Singing Your Own Song

USING THE MIND-BODY CONNECTION TO ENHANCE YOUR HEALTH

by

Susan Dinklage Multer

dp
DISTINCTIVE PUBLISHING

Library of Congress Cataloging-in-Publication Data
Multer, Susan Dinklage, 1942 —
Singing your own song : using the mind-body connection to enhance your health / Susan Dinklage Multer.
   p.   cm.
Includes bibliographical references
ISBN 0-942963-51-2: $7.95
1. Medicine, Psychosomatic.   2. Mind and body.
3. Psychoneuroimmunology.   4. Breast—Cancer   I. Title
RC49.M835   1994
616'.001'9—dc20
                                              94-23113
                                                   CIP

Cover design by Chris Pearl
Typesetting by Mary Bredbenner

Distinctive books are available at special discounts when purchased in bulk for premiums and sales promotions as well as for fund-raising or educational use. Special Editions or book excerpts can also be created to specification. For details, contact the Special Sales Director at the address below.

dp

DISTINCTIVE PUBLISHING
P.O. Box 17868
Plantation, Florida 33318-7868

Manufactured in the United States of America

Dedicated with love

to

my mother

Elizabeth Payne Bullard Dinklage

Each person is seen as having a special song to sing; a special rhythm to beat out in terms of his acting, reacting, relating and creating. When he sings his own song, he experiences a zest for life, an enjoyment of life, and a meaning in life...In most cases, the patient's despair arises out of the fact that he or she has not been singing his or her unique song. They have tried to sing other people's songs all their lives, and the effort has brought them only frustration and self-contempt. Nothing can be more important for them than to discover their own particular song and learn to project it loudly and clearly.

You Can Fight For Your Life
Lawrence LeShan, 1977

Contents

APPRECIATION vii

FOREWORD ix

INTRODUCTION xi

Part I. FIGHTING THE TIGER WITHIN 1
    1. THAT SPECIAL SUNSHINE 3
    2. TIPPING THE ICEBERG 7

Part II. DISCOVERING THE MIND-BODY CONNECTION . 11
    3. ANCIENT TO MODERN EVIDENCE 13
    4. SCIENTIFIC EXPLANATION 17
        Fight or Flight Response 17
        Chronic Stress Syndrome 19
        New Directions in Psychotherapy 19
        Psychoneuroimmunology 22
        The Meaning of Stress 24

PART III. SINGING YOUR OWN SONG 27
    5. DEVELOPING A POSITIVE OUTLOOK 29
        Expectations 29
        Visualization 30
        The Will to Live 31
        Expression of Negative Feelings 33
    6. TAKING CHARGE 37
        Participation in Decision Making 37
        Saying No 38
        Developing a Support System 39
        Setting Goals 42

7. EATING WITHOUT GUILT 45
   Failure of the Four Food Groups 45
   Politics of the Food Pyramid 47
   Diet for Good Health 48
   When "Good" Can be Hazardous to Your Health. 49
   Alternatives to Deprivation 50

8. KEEPING FIT 53
   Aerobic Exercise 53
   Cardiovascular Benefits 54
   Psychological Benefits 54
   Weight Control 55
   Longevity 55
   When Walking is Not an Option 56
   Perseverance 57

9. TAKING TIME OUT 59
   Progressive Muscle Relaxation 59
   Deep Breathing 60
   Meditation 60
   Hobbies 61
   Pets 62
   Music 64

10. LIFTING THE SPIRIT 65
    Laughter 66
    Love 69
    Hope 69
    Faith 69
    Forgiveness 70
    Wisdom 71

CONCLUSION 73

REFERENCES 75

INDEX 81

Appreciation

$\mathcal{F}$AMILY AND FRIENDS, as well as health professionals, have been my teachers regarding the relationship between emotions and health. Several have encouraged or inspired me to write about it. In the chronological order in which they influenced me, I sincerely thank the following:

- Helen Bullard, whose determination to live (in spite of medical odds against it) I did not understand as a child, but do now
- Dr. Frank Gump, whose kindness and caring epitomized the ideal doctor-patient relationship and whose insight inspired confidence and hope
- Ruth Cetrulo, who first taught me the importance of attitude and expectations with regard to health
- Helen Dinklage, who introduced me to visualization
- Dr. Louis Schwartz, whose sensitivity and skill allayed my fears of radiation and helped in healing
- Pat Thompson, who said from the beginning that I had something important to write
- Jakob Steinberg, who introduced me to Carl Simonton's work
- Myrna Rose, who introduced me to Bernie Siegel's work
- Norman Cousins, Lawrence LeShan, Bernie Siegel and Carl Simonton, whose books helped me immensely and enabled me to help others
- Bill Stockfield, who shared his computer
- Ruth Gruber and Bonnie Yannie, who dared to love someone who already had cancer
- Bob Newman, Ossy Walker and Ruth Wilson, who are exceptional survivors
- students in my classes who are living with rheumatoid arthritis, cancer, diabetes, lupus and multiple schlerosis
- Arthur Baird, Edna Carter and Phil McHenry, whose lives touched and inspired us
- my husband, Gray, whose love, support and encouragement from the beginning have enabled me to complete this project

$\mathcal{F}$oreword

$\mathcal{I}$N THE FIELD OF HEALTH PSYCHOLOGY we recognize that a new definition of health has emerged over the last twenty years. It is the view that health is the presence of positive well-being rather than merely the absence of disease. Six different areas have been identified as significant in order to increase the likelihood of positive well-being, or state of wellness. Thus positive changes in these areas can reduce the likelihood of illness. The areas are physical fitness and nutrition, emotional wellness, occupational satisfaction, spirituality, family/social/community involvement, and intellectual stimulation.

Formerly, infectious diseases were the leading cause of death in the United States; now cardiovascular disease and cancer are most common. Chronic and progressive, these diseases are often related to lifestyle. Thus there are behavioral changes we could make that might enhance our health. This book offers a comprehensive yet common sense approach to learning the steps necessary for those types of lifestyle interventions.

In my clinical practice and teaching I have done extensive work with traumatic stress reactions to disaster, physical injury and medical illness. This work includes disaster mental health services provided to civilian casualties as well as to emergency responders such as law enforcement officers, firefighters, and rescue squad members who in their line of duty are exposed to events which lead to the experience of Critical Incident Stress.

In treating victims of traumatic stress I make the same kinds of recommendations offered in this book, to civilians or emergency responders alike. The impact of traumatic events has repercussions in the cognitive, affective, physiological and behavioral spheres. The strategies offered here are excellent guidelines for us all to follow in order to maintain or regain our health. Without doing so, we are at significant risk.

Prolonged stress, whether stemming from despair over loss of a loved one or anger at being treated unfairly, has a profound affect physiologically as well as psychologically. It puts the person in a chronic state of fight or flight which is so disruptive that the body is no longer able to function efficiently and effectively. Specific changes in the nervous system and endocrine system have the impact of reducing the immunocompetence, thereby increasing the likelihood of susceptibility to, and the actual development of, chronic illness.

A dramatic example is found in the adrenal and thymus glands. Unresolved feelings of anxiety or loss of control create such a demand for adrenaline that the adrenal glands actually expand in order to meet the increased need when one is in a constant (relatively speaking) fight or flight state. This expansion has an adverse affect upon the thymus gland which produces the T-cell and B-cell leukocytes. These are the white blood cells which serve as an early detection, early warning, early search-and-destroy mechanism to eliminate invaders such as cancer cells. The more the adrenal gland expands, the more the thymus gland shrinks and the fewer killer cells will be produced. Thus long-term, unabated stress can negatively impact the body's regulatory mechanisms and compromise the effectiveness of our immune system.

When I first read *Sing Your Own Song*, I was impressed with the author's recognition of the complexity of illness and her openness to the convergence of multiple factors contributing to health. Only someone with a multidisciplinary background could bring together the mind-body relationship so well. Only someone who has survived a life-threatening illness could write from the perspective she does. This book provides an elegant rationale for lifestyle changes that optimize the quality of life. Susan Dinklage Multer is an exceptional teacher who makes it her paramount personal mission to share these insights with the rest of the world.

My pleasure is in having piqued the author's original musing that led to her research and self-discovery which culminated in the writing of this book. It is an important combination of personal experience and scientific data that is well documented and truly insightful. In keeping with today's strong public interest in health promotion, this is an essential manual that needed to be written.

Jakob Steinberg, Ph.D.

Professor of Psychology
Fairleigh Dickinson University, Madison New Jersey

Trauma Response Coordinator
New Jersey Psychological Association

Introduction

ONE DOESN'T HAVE TO BE A SCIENTIST to have observed over the years that some people who smoke a pack of cigarettes a day don't get lung cancer and others who have never smoked in their life do. Likewise, some business executives in very high stress situations don't develop heart disease, while others in the leisure of retirement do. The unanswered question is why?

Equally puzzling is the fact that strict vegetarians can die at an early age and others who eat a high fat diet live a long life. In like manner, some joggers never make it to fifty, while some sedentary people live into their nineties. With all due respect to the excellent, in-depth research on the causes and treatment of our two most significant life-threatening illnesses (heart disease and cancer), incidence remains high and cures are exceptional.

Perhaps this paradox exists because a very important element has been overlooked. In ancient Chinese and Greek culture there was awareness of a relationship between emotions and illness. It was still being investigated as recently as the nineteenth century in Europe and the United States, but it later came to be discredited or ignored in the West.

Early twentieth century research basically focused on genetics or environment. Given the statistics showing that family history of cancer and heart disease is significant, it is logical to look for genes to provide an explanation. But why do some members of a particular family get sick and others stay well? Likewise, much work has been done to show that substances such as asbestos and PCB's can be carcinogenic, but all workers exposed to them do not develop cancer. Even with regard to diet, although third world countries consume little fat and have a low incidence of heart disease, a low fat diet does not guarantee protection. It is obvious that other factors are involved.

In recent years there has been a growing interest in the influence of the mind, positively or negatively, on our health. It is called the mind-body connection. Unfortunately, some aspects have been taken out of context or exaggerated, with the end result that the idea has sometimes been mistakenly considered a New Age philosophy of mind control. Nothing could be further from the truth. We cannot control our health. What we can do is recognize that in addition to the obvious influences such as heredity, enviromental exposure and diet, there is a hidden factor that can be significant: our emotions.

What some physicians suspected for centuries has now been confirmed through scientific studies. Long term, unabated negative feelings such as anger or depression directly affect our immune system and make us more susceptible to illness. Thus the ancient question of whether there is a relationship between emotions and health has been answered with a resounding, "Yes!"

The purpose of this book is to introduce readers to this subject and at the same time enable them to apply its principles to themselves and to their students, clients or patients. Chapters 1 and 2 briefly describe my discovery of the relationship between emotions and health during my experience with cancer ten years ago; Chapters 3 and 4 highlight the historical evidence of and explanation for the mind-body connection. The main emphasis, however, is on what we can do to help ourselves. Chapters 5 through 10 delineate six areas in which we can make significant changes in everyday life which can help free our immune system to function normally, thereby enhancing our health.

Therein lies the hope, the opportunity and the challenge.

PART I

Fighting the Tiger Within

1

That Special Sunshine

IT WAS EASTER 1985. It had been a glorious day, with sunny skies and the fragrance of flowers in bloom. The visual beauty was surpassed only by the sound of the organist at Basking Ridge Presbyterian Church, playing Widor's "Toccata" from the Fifth Symphony, the magnificent piece we had chosen for the recessional at our wedding, years before.

We had gone to bed early and were cuddling. As my husband embraced me, he said, "What's this?" thinking that he felt something unusual in my left breast.

"Just normal tissue," I replied, pushing his hand away and adding flippantly, "No lumps allowed tonight!" The mood was not broken and we made love.

The following evening my husband reminded me to do a breast check, and there it was, a hard, round lump, right at the surface.

"This is it," I said, as if I'd known it were coming.

Twice I'd had lumps elsewhere which turned out to be swollen lymph nodes. This was different. All I could think of was whether, when and how to tell my father. It seemed too cruel, since he had already suffered through my mother's two mastectomies and death some thirty-five years earlier.

Ironically, the mammogram the next day was negative, but the ultrasound indicated that the mass was dense and warranted further evaluation. The surgeon recommended by my internist used the old-fashioned, one-step approach: put the patient in the hospital, remove the lump under general anesthesia, do a frozen section analysis, and, if it's malignant, remove more tissue and lymph nodes. I told him to schedule the surgery as soon as possible but also asked the name of another surgeon in order to get a second opinion. He recommended the chief of surgery at the same hospital.

When I went for the second opinion, I was offered the option of having the lump removed in the doctor's office, under local anesthetic. After analysis, more surgery could be scheduled if needed. The second doctor indicated an advantage to the two-step procedure: the analysis was more in-depth than the frozen section, and it would give more information about the specific type of cancer.

Suddenly I questioned the wisdom of what I was doing: (1) going to general surgeons rather than those specializing in cancer, (2) consulting two from the same facility, and (3) choosing my local community hospital. So I cancelled the pending surgery and made an appointment with Dr. Frank E. Gump, who was Chief of Breast Surgery at Columbia Presbyterian Medical Center, where he had worked for thirty years.

Gump was as compassionate as he was skilled. Gray-haired, kind and gentle, he answered my long list of questions without irritation or ridicule. He was up on the latest research, quoting a study published in the *New England Journal of Medicine* that month indicating that lumpectomy patients had as good survival rates after five years as those who had had mastectomies. Since my lump was small and new (it had not been evident in my complete physical three months before), he said I was a good candidate for lumpectomy.

Sensing my fear of radiation, Gump acknowledged that it could conceivably contribute to new cancer in about twenty years, but he pointed out that without it, a reoccurrence could happen in two or three years simply because the surgery hadn't removed all the cells. His calm logic convinced me that if I did have cancer, I should have the radiation.

I was totally taken by surprise when he offered to do needle aspiration. "But I thought that could give false negatives!" I blurted out.

He acknowledged that it could, but he went on to say that the pathology department at Columbia was so sophisticated that about 90% of the breast malignancies are found this way, the least invasive method possible. Reports that do come back negative are questioned, and then a biopsy is performed.

Once again I felt reassured. I also felt relieved to learn that instead of just hearing a third opinion, I could get action on the spot. It had, after all, been twelve days since the lump had been found. The needle aspiration was quick and almost painless, as was the report of the malignancy the next morning by telephone. I remember my response: "I'm so glad to find it out this way." I'd had no surgery, no anesthetic, no hospitalization.

Unfortunately, Dr. Gump was leaving the next day for a lecture tour in Europe. Not wanting to wait two weeks, I asked for a referral. He suggested a colleague at CPMC or Dr. Befeler at Overlook Hospital in Summit, New Jersey. I saw both and chose the latter. Gump had told me that Befeler was a "pioneer in lumpectomy" and used a technique that could prevent any lingering numbness. (It did.)

As the day of surgery neared, I wondered if having a masectomy would have been a better choice. I wasn't sure about my rationale for questioning the procedure I'd chosen. Was it that the more aggressive surgery might be more likely to get all the cancer cells, or was I just wishing to avoid radiation? In desperation, the day before surgery I called a doctor in Boston whose name I had read as having done lumpectomies for a long time. Somehow I got past the receptionist and spoke with the doctor in person to ask my simple, but profound, question: did he have any patients who had had lumpectomies ten or fifteen years ago who were still alive? He did.

That was all I needed to hear. I went for surgery, confident and optimistic. I was home in two days and hanging up laundry in five. The next week we got the report that the lymph nodes were negative. My husband started calling me Mrs. Clean.

Yet I still faced the hurdle of radiation. Back at work ten days after the surgery, I commented to a colleague, Ruth Cetrulo, that I was more concerned about the radiation than the cancer. Realizing how ridiculous that sounded, I explained, "Not to minimize cancer, but my mother died of it just before I turned seven, and all my adult life I've known that, statistically, my chances of getting it were higher than others'."

I shall never forget Ruth's response. Looking me straight in the eye, she said, "Susan, my mother died when I was a child, too, but all my adult life I've told myself I'll never get cancer."

I was shocked. How could an intelligent person believe that one's thoughts could affect one's health? Not wanting to offend my friend, I smiled and nodded politely and continued the conversation in a different direction. Little did I know how wise Ruth was and how much I had yet to learn.

My immediate concern was the 35 radiation treatments I was facing. The issue was not pain, but unknown side effects. Knowing my concerns, my aunt spoke to me of a friend whose son, an anti-nuclear activist, needed to undergo radiation. He overcame his fears by picturing the radiation killing the cancer cells. I decided to try it.

The radiation was done at Overlook. The first day, as the machine buzzed at me, I thought of lava from a volcano, smothering things as it flowed down the slopes. The only problem was, I knew it killed everything it touched. So I modified the idea and decided to personify the beam coming out of the machine. I called it my special sunshine.

Each day as I lay on the table, I would say (in my mind), "Good morning, sunshine!" Then I'd say something like, "Get in there and kill those cancer cells. Get the teeny weeny ones that nobody even knows are there." Or, "I'm glad I'm living in the 1980s in the U.S., where this technology is available." Or whatever. I never planned it beforehand or thought about it afterwards, but it was incredibly effective. Instead of dreading the experience, I was actually reassured by it.

A friend surprised me later by asking how many treatments I had left. It was as though she expected me to be counting, "One down, thirty-four to go," from the first day through the seven weeks. It was not like that at all. The procedure was painless, I suffered no side effects except tiredness, and the staff was as sensitive in human relations as it was skilled in technique. All in all, it was a very positive experience. I went straight from the last treatment to the airport, where I caught a flight to Los Angeles and then went on to New Zealand for vacation. The cancer was behind me.

So I thought.

2

Tipping the Iceberg

THE FOLLOWING WINTER our friend Jakob Steinberg, Professor of Psychology at Fairleigh Dickinson University, learned tha' I had had cancer. He told me that researchers had found that many who get cancer have suffered a loss, such as a loved one or a job, before developing the illness. He wondered if I had. I said no, but that I'd been under the greatest stress of my life, struggling through science courses in graduate school at age 43. He surmised that my studying hard and not doing as well as expected brought a feeling of loss of control. He seemed to be trying to make parts of my life fit into a theory in which he believed, and, frankly, I didn't buy it.

The next month my husband was awarded a Fulbright grant to teach in Germany during the 1986-87 school year. Consequently I requested a leave of absence without pay from the school district in which I was a social worker. The Board of Education met, discussed my request and tabled it. That's when I knew I was in trouble.

The next day I went to the Superintendent to find out what had happened. He said the Board was simply worried about setting a bad precedent. After all, I had already been granted two such leaves in ten years of employment, in order to assist my husband on other research ventures. "But don't worry," he said reassuringly. "You can just resign and then reapply when you return."

Delighted, I left his office and headed happily down the hall. Within minutes, however, my hope faded as I realized I'd have no legal right to the job later. Furthermore, I might be in the awkward position of competing with a social worker who was less experienced and therefore could be paid a lower salary (which would be very appealing to the Board). The thought of having to fight for my job brought to the surface the pain I'd been repressing for three years.

By the time I reached the principal's office I was so angry I blurted out, "If the Board thinks I'm going to come back begging for my job after what they did to me three years ago, they don't know Susan Multer!" As I drove home, I vividly recalled and relived what had happened that horrible year.

*It was 1983. We were in Antigua, for my husband's Sabbatical. I was on leave from my school district, and it was the time of year that contracts were coming out for the following fall. Because of declining enrollment, some staff positions had already been reduced, and I anticipated that this year the social work position would be cut from three days to two. When the letter arrived, however, I discovered that my position had been reduced to **one** day per week.*

Surprised as I was, in typical Susan fashion I signed and returned the paper, merely thinking, "Things must be worse than I thought." I meant in the district; in fact, the words were prophetic for me. Upon return I learned that while my position had been decreased by two days, the psychologist's had been increased by one.

I was FURIOUS! My options were to go to the Board, the newspaper, or the NJEA (New Jersey Education Association) to point out publicly that the extra work the psychologist was going to do was work for which I was equally qualified. However, I rationalized that even if I won the battle, I would lose the war in the sense that my working relationship with the administration and staff would be ruined. I didn't think it was worth it. So in my usual, submissive style, I decided to grin and bear it.

It wasn't easy. Every week in my one day on the job, I was reminded of my marginal status. I never knew what had happened the rest of the week in the classroom or on the playground, let alone what had been talked about in the teachers' room. When a parent called and asked for counseling, the case had to be assigned to the psychologist because the social worker wasn't there often enough for follow-up.

One day I discovered new triplicate memo pads on which were printed the name of the middle school principal and the school psychologist, but not the school social worker. This time I was absolutely LIVID! I immediately ventilated my anger to the elementary school principal and the speech therapist, but that didn't suffice. The next thing I knew I was headed down the hall to the Superintendent's office. Seeing his door open and no one in conference, I walked right past his secretary, barged into his office, and asked if I could speak with him for a minute. "Look at this!" I exclaimed, as I handed him the memo pad. "Either the psychologist's name should not be on it or the social worker's should be. It isn't right! It isn't fair!" I then heard these words spill out of my mouth: "I'm tired of being treated like SHIT!"

Unruffled, he said he didn't have anything to do with the memo; it was ordered by the middle school principal.

"I know that," I said emphatically. "That's why I'm coming to you. I want someone at the top to know how I feel!" I stormed out of his office, leaving three secretaries speechless.

It is important for the reader to remember that I was recalling this incident three years after it happened. Just thinking about it made me so angry that my hands got hot and sweaty and my heart beat faster. At long last I realized its significance. To have acted so inappropriately, so unprofessionally, so out of character for me meant that there was much more beneath the surface. My brief explosion had been only the tip of the iceberg; the rest was still down deep.

Then I remembered Jakob Steinberg's recent question about a loss prior to my cancer. I hadn't lost my job, but I'd lost two thirds of it, which was worse because of the constant reminder of being a nobody. I had lost my *raison d'etre*, my reason for being, in the school district. Though I'd never heard a word about the mind-body connection, I instinctively understood that my bottled up anger, resentment and jealousy had something to do with my cancer.

As I paced the floor at home thinking of what I should have said to the school board three years earlier, I realized that I was in the unique position of having an excuse to speak to that same group of people now on another subject: my request for a leave of absence. The Superintendent gave me permission to go to the closed session and speak on my own behalf.

For two weeks I planned and rehearsed what I would say. The night of the meeting I gave a brief, four-point presentation regarding the uniqueness and value of my early intervention programs in the classroom. I asked if they had any questions; they did not. Then I said there was one question they might ask after I left the room, namely, why not deny the leave to avoid public criticism for granting me another one. Then I could simply reapply upon return.

At that point I changed my tone of voice and whole demeanor, looking the five board members in the eye one by one, as I "*socked it to them*" with the single sentence and poignant pauses I'd been rehearsing for days: "Anyone thinking that...has no idea...how devastated and humiliated I was...both personally and professionally...when three years ago this board cut my job by two thirds...something which has never been done to anyone else in this district...in order to increase the time of another member of the child study team...to do work that I am equally qualified to do."

Resuming my polite, professional stance, I concluded, "I'm excited about what I do in this district, and I want to come back and continue. If you feel the same way, you'll vote for this leave of absence. Thank you."

As I headed down the hall I felt absolutely ecstatic. "It doesn't matter whether I get the leave of absence," I said to my husband. "I feel relieved! I feel reprieved! I feel like I've had my day in court...my say in court...I feel like I've gotten off my chest..."

I couldn't finish the sentence because the symbolism was so significant. I'd bottled up anger, resentment and jealousy for years and then developed a breast lump. Just now I'd finally expressed the anger and hurt to the people who had caused it, and I felt as though the weight of the world had been lifted. There was definitely a connection. I lay awake that night, high with hope about my new insight and with anticipation of learning more. I called Jakob the next morning and asked the name of the book he had so highly recommended.

It was Simonton's *Getting Well Again*. Within a few pages I learned that most of the cancer patients with whom they had worked had experienced a significant loss in the two years before development of the disease. So had I. Many of their patients had used visualization successfully to help with their treatment. So had I. The philosophy behind their program was succinctly and profoundly stated as follows:

"Everyone participates in his or her own health or illness at all times...It is our central premise that an illness is not purely a physical problem but rather a problem of the whole person, that it includes not only body but mind and emotions. We believe that emotional and mental states play a significant role both in *susceptibility* to disease, including cancer, and in *recovery* from all disease" (Simonton, *et al.*, 1978).

That was my introduction to the mind-body connection. Fascinated with the idea and filled with hope, I read on and on.

PART II

Discovering the Mind – Body Connection

3 —————————————

Ancient To
Modern Evidence

*T*HE IDEA IS NOT NEW. For centuries the Chinese have believed that thoughts and emotions affect health. Their early morning activities in public parks across the country demonstrate their belief that centering themselves and concentrating their mind can free their vital energy, or force of life, called "Chi" (Moyers, 1993). The ancient Greeks also believed in the mind-body connection. As early as 500 B.C., Socrates is reported to have philosophized, "There is no illness of the body apart from the mind." The physician Galen observed and recorded in 180 A.D. that melancholy women were more prone to cancer than happy ones. In the wisdom attributed to King Solomon it is phrased this way: "A cheerful heart is good medicine, but a downcast spirit dries up the bones" (Proverbs 17:22). Although the words have changed over time, the concept remains the same: our emotions can affect our health.

A review of the medical literature by Kowal (1955) and LeShan (1959) revealed many references in the 18th and 19th centuries to the influence of the mind on the body. A sampling will show its significance.

The British surgeon Richard Guy, after stating that women are especially subject to cancer after suffering "such Disasters in Life as occasion much trouble and Grief," goes on to give two specific examples:

Case 1: Mrs. Emerson, upon the Death of their Daughter, underwent great Affliction, and perceived her Breast to swell, which soon after grew painful; at last it broke out in a most inveterate Cancer, which consumed a great Part of it in a short Time. She had always enjoyed a perfect state of health.

Case 2: The Wife of a mate of a Ship (who was taken some Time ago by the French and put in Prison) was thereby so much affected, that her Breast began to swell, and soon after broke out in a desperate Cancer which had proceeded so far that I could not undertake her case. She had never before had any Complaint in her Breast (Guy, 1759).

Similar observations were made by other physicians in other places. By the 19th century it was well known that losses or other negative events in life often preceded the onset of illness even though there was no explanation of how there could be any connection between the two. Nevertheless, the potential significance was noted.

The French physician Amussat stated the concept very simply: "This idea seems true to me that cancer is caused most frequently by grief, and by all the physical and moral disturbances which are its result" (Amussat, 1854).

Sir James Paget, the world-renowned British surgeon and pathologist, was more specific:

> *The cases are so frequent in which deep anxiety, deferred hope and disappointment, are quickly followed by the growth or increase of cancer that we can hardly doubt that mental depression is a weighty addition to the other influences that favour the development of the cancerous constitution* (Paget, 1870).

But how? Without even the insight of psychoanalysis, let alone the more recent revelations regarding the mind-body connection, the incidents could only be considered sheer coincidence. Worse yet, the investigations could be written off as self-fulfilling prophecies on the part of the investigators. In other words, they had a hypothesis and were looking for pieces of people's lives that supported the theory.

It was the British surgeon Herbert Snow who first gathered statistical data on this subject. According to LeShan (1959), in three books Snow espoused his theories and summarized his findings, which included histories of 250 successive inpatients and outpatients at the London Cancer Hospital on one occasion and

140 breast cancer patients on another. He found that in the vast majority of cases the illness had been preceded by a significant "trouble," such as loss of a loved one, hard work or deprivation (Snow, 1870, 1883, 1893). Yet he knew the idea was not universally accepted. He profoundly concluded:

> *I am well aware that depression of mind as a forerunner of cancer has been noticed by numerous observers...Yet I scarcely think they have assigned to their observations the weight it deserves; nor, so far as my limited knowledge goes, has it materially influenced medical thought, or the view held by the bulk of our profession. And even among those who have described it, the field of vision would seem to have been obscured by false considerations of hereditary tendency, and by other injurious theories* (Snow, 1883).

How right Snow was. Even his statistics could be ignored. After all, the fact that A precedes B does not mean that A caused B. Even with statistically significant numbers, it is merely a correlation, and correlation doesn't necessarily prove cause and effect.

A contemporary of Snow's was the U.S. surgeon Willard Parker, who was writing a book about his 53 years of experience with 397 cases of breast cancer. He, too, had noted the influence of the mind on the body and approached the subject through a series of questions:

> *Now can anxiety be a predisposing cause? Will a long period of care, trouble, and sorrow alone disturb the balance between the nervous and cellular elements, so as to make the latter take on an abnormal, a cancerous, development? It is more than probable; but can it be demonstrated? Perhaps not; but must we on that account reject the probability? Are we justified in rejecting every hypothesis which cannot be placed upon a demonstrated basis?* (Parker, 1885)

Justified or not, the majority of the medical profession did reject the idea. To them it seemed inconceivable that one's mind, emotions, personality or coping style had anything to do with illness. Even with the development of psychoanalytic theory and Freud's success in alleviating or sometimes eliminating physical symptoms through psychological intervention, the idea was not well respected in his time.

According to Kowol (1955), there were two schools of thought about cancer in the 19th century: (1) cancer was a local, cellular problem, or (2) it was a general, constitutional one. By the turn of the century the local theory dominated and led to a focus on treatment at the local site. As methods of surgery and types of anesthetics improved, followed by radiation and eventually chemotherapy, the earlier investigations and theories were forgotten. The idea of a mind-body connection fell into disrepute and lay like an unfinished puzzle in an attic, waiting for the missing pieces to be found.

4

Scientific Explanation

Fight or Flight Response

IT WASN'T UNTIL THE 1920s that the physiologist Walter Cannon did the animal studies that provided the missing link. He discovered that when animals were frightened, their bodies automatically responded with changes. They did so by means of the sympathetic or autonomic nervous system, which regulates body processes that go on without our thinking about them. Examples include beating of the heart, circulation of the blood, and breathing. In the laboratory experiments when the animals were faced with danger, their hearts beat faster, respiration rate increased, pupils of the eyes dilated, and blood was redirected away from the skin to the muscles. The additional oxygen delivered in the process gave the animal extra strength and endurance to either fight or run away from the source of danger.

This phenomenon, which Cannon described in his book *The Wisdom of the Body* (1939), later came to be known as the "fight or flight" response. It applies to humans, too. Imagine, for example, a caveman suddenly approached by a tiger. He has only two means of survival: 1) fight and kill (or severely wound) the beast or 2) outrun him. The body is miraculously programmed for survival, and the physiological changes noted above make it possible.

We have all heard of ordinary people performing extraordinary tasks when someone's life depended on it. Note the mother who lifts a car when her child is under it or the teenager who lifts a fallen tree to free his father. The brain signals the sympathetic nervous system to "pull out all stops," thereby enabling superhuman behavior for the moment. When the crisis ends, the body returns to equilibrium.

The significance of Cannon's work should be emphasized. His studies proved that emotions such as fear or panic cause measurable physiological changes. What they did not show was how that fight or flight response relates to illness.

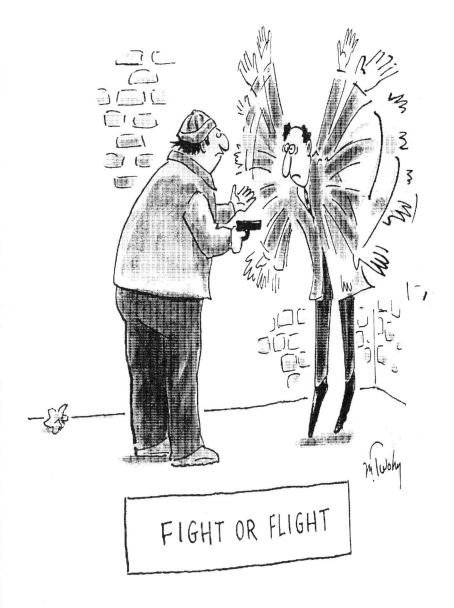

FIGHT OR FLIGHT

Chronic Stress Syndrome

It was Hans Selye, endocrinologist at the University of Montreal and former student of Cannon's, who raised the question of what happens when the stress is not the result of a temporary crisis but rather a long-term problem. His studies led to the realization that the sympathetic nervous system responds to the "alarm" signal whether the source of alarm is a wild tiger, an unfaithful spouse, or an unfair job situation. Since it is not socially acceptable to slap one's boss in the face, there is no resolution to the problem, and the nervous system remains "on alert." Physiological changes take place, including overproduction of certain neurochemicals which subsequently have a negative effect upon our health.

Selye initially named this concept the "general adaptation syndrome" in 1946. Today we call it chronic stress. It is what I mean by "the tiger within," in the title of Part I of this book. With the publication of Selye's book *The Stress of Life* in 1956, the old question of a mind-body connection resurfaced, this time not to be ignored. As more studies were done, the idea gained credibility. It was given extra impetus in 1959 by Dr. Eugene P. Pendergrass, President of the American Cancer Society, when he said:

> *Anyone who has had an extensive experience in the treatment of cancer is aware that there are great differences among patients....There is solid evidence that the course of the disease in general is affected by emotional distress....it is my sincere hope that we can widen the quest to include the distinct possibility that within one's mind is a power capable of exerting forces which can either enhance or inhibit the progress of this disease* (quoted in Simonton, *et al.*, 1978).

New Directions in Psychotherapy

One who seriously pursued that quest was psychologist Lawrence LeShan. Wondering why some people exposed to a carcinogen get cancer and others don't, he began studying the life situations and personalities of cancer patients in the 1950s. Common elements he found included lack of purpose or direction, inability to express anger on one's own behalf, and loss of a meaningful relationship. Often the patient had lost a parent during childhood.

LeShan's early research is summarized in his book *You Can Fight for Your Life* (1977). With a significant degree of success, he used his findings to counsel patients to change their attitude and coping skills. Instead of asking what was wrong, he focused on what was right by asking questions like, "What are your special ways of being, relating, acting, creating?" and, "What is blocking their expression?" (LeShan, 1977). In this way he helped people free themselves to be who they wanted to be. Further refinement and results of his work are found in his later book, *Cancer As a Turning Point* (1989).

It was psychiatrist George Solomon who published an early paper on emotions, immunity and disease (Solomon and Moos, 1964) and coined the word psychoimmunology, long before people understood its implications. His work contributed greatly to the field which later came to be called psychoneuroimmunology. After many years of working with patients who had life-threatening illnesses, he identified and named another significant concept: the immunosuppression-prone personality (Solomon, 1985).

A physician who pursued a similar line of research in the 1960s was radiation oncologist O. Carl Simonton. Intrigued with the fact that some patients with good prognoses died soon and some with poor prognoses lived unusually long, he asked patients in the latter category what they thought was the reason for their outliving medical expectations. Their spontaneous answers were simple but profound: "I have small children to raise," or, "There's no one to take over my business." Capitalizing on their will to live and using techniques from biofeedback to visualize regression of their cancer, Simonton created a program that has brought help and health to hundreds of patients directly and many more indirectly, through training other health professionals here and abroad. The philosophy and program are described in *Getting Well Again* (Simonton, et al., 1978) and further elaborated in *The Healing Journey* (Simonton, et al., 1992).

When these (and other) investigators were working successfully with cancer patients in the 1950s and early '60s, they were showing that the mind does affect the body. Yet they still did not know exactly how. Then, one by one, different researchers discovered different parts of the answer. Important examples include finding blood vessels that link the hypothalamus (part of the brain) to the pituitary gland (Scharrer and Scharrer, 1963), locating receptors on immune cells that can receive messages from the brain (Pert, *et al.*, 1973), and demonstrating that the brain talks to the body via peptides (Guillemin, 1978; Schally, 1978).

Both being former students of Hans Selye, Guillemin (in Houston) and Schally (in New Orleans) independently made the discoveries for which they were jointly awarded the 1977 Nobel Prize in physiology or medicine (Justice, 1988).

It was Robert Ader and Nathan Cohen at the University of Rochester School of Medicine who performed a landmark study showing that expectations can affect the immune response (Ader and Cohen, 1975). Since the original animal studies, the concept has been used clinically to treat an adolescent who had been suffering from lupus, an autoimmune disease. Using taste and smell for conditioning, the team (physicians, psychologists, patient and family) successfully influenced the immune response, bringing measureable benefits that have lasted for eight years (Moyers, 1993).

An extremely important discovery made by David Felten, also from the University of Rochester School of Medicine, occurred when he identified nerve endings in cells of the immune system (Felten, *et al.*, 1985). This finding so contradicted the long-accepted belief that the immune system was independent that Felten and his colleagues were initially reluctant to talk about it. Since then, he has written:

> *Just as the physical world of rainbows, lightning, and stars was not understood in the centuries before modern physics and astronomy, so also the more elusive and complex aspects of the human mind are not understood at present....Can we afford to ignore the role of emotions, hope, the will to live, the power of human warmth and contact, just because they are difficult to investigate scientifically and our ignorance is so overwhelming?*
> (Felten, 1991)

No, we cannot. These studies (and others) have provided the missing pieces of the puzzle: scientific proof that the brain communicates directly with the immune system. Thus the ancient question of whether there is a relationship between emotions and health has been answered with a resounding, "Yes!"

Psychoneuroimmunology (PNI)

The new name for this old field of study is psychoneuroimmunology (PNI). It involves the interaction of the nervous system (which includes the brain), the endocrine system (which produces the hormones), and the immune system. The classic text on psychoneuroimmunology was published by Ader, et al., in 1981; the first world conference on the subject was held in 1988.

Two important means of communication are neurotransmitters and hormones. Both send messages to various parts of the body, thereby stimulating or inhibiting a multitude of processes. A neurotransmitter acts very quickly, bringing a message almost instantly from the cell that secretes it to the targeted one. Hormones take more time (minutes or even hours) to respond.

The word neurotransmitter was chosen because originally we thought that these chemical substances only came from the nervous system. We now know that the pathway of communication is "bi-directional," i.e., the immune system also influences and communicates with the neural and endocrine systems (Ader, et al., 1991).

The hormone with which most people are familiar is insulin. When blood levels of glucose (also called blood sugar) are too high, a signal is sent to the pancreas to produce insulin, which then stimulates the liver and muscle cells to take excess glucose from the blood stream. Another well-known hormone is adrenaline, or epinephrine, which is produced by the adrenal gland when the organism is subjected to stress. Our understanding of this process is evident in the common phrase, "My adrenaline is up."

So why is that a problem? Isn't it exactly what the body is supposed to do? Yes, in short term crises. But long-term, unabated stress causes excess production of neurotransmitters and stress hormones, with the end result that the immune system is compromised. Then it cannot fight off foreign agents whether viruses or cancer cells. Then we become susceptible to illness.

A complete discussion of our immune system would constitute a book in itself. For our purposes we merely need to know that there are many levels of resistance and defense. Whether the "invaders" enter through the mouth, the nose, the skin or genetic mutation, we have an array of forces to stop them. These include, but are not limited to: macrophages (scavenger cells), natural killer cells (special white blood cells that have a major role in fighting viruses and cancer), antibodies (proteins which attack foreign agents with which they are familiar), cytotoxic T cells (made by the thymus gland to fight invaders), and helper T cells which are involved in stimulating the activity of most of the elements just described). See Figure 4-1 for details.

YOUR DEPARTMENT OF DEFENSE. The body is an amazing mechanism. Once invaded—by fungi, parasites, bacteria, or viruses—a complex series of reactions takes place to defeat the enemy. Pictured here are the principal players of the immune system. Not shown are the many proteins, including the interferons and interleukins, which also help drive the immune system.

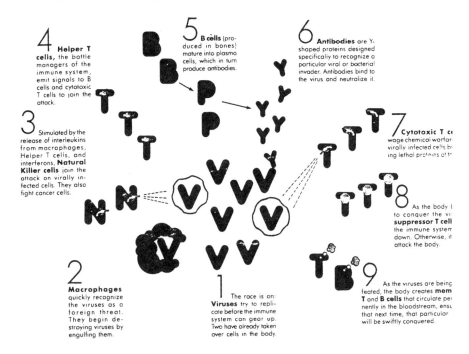

4 **Helper T cells,** the battle managers of the immune system, emit signals to B cells and cytotoxic T cells to join the attack.

5 **B cells** (produced in bones) mature into plasma cells, which in turn produce antibodies.

6 **Antibodies** are Y-shaped proteins designed specifically to recognize a particular viral or bacterial invader. Antibodies bind to the virus and neutralize it.

3 Stimulated by the release of interleukins from macrophages, Helper T cells, and interferons, **Natural Killer cells** join the attack on virally infected cells. They also fight cancer cells.

7 **Cytotoxic T ce** wage chemical warfar virally infected cells by ing lethal proteins at th

8 As the body b to conquer the vi **suppressor T cell** the immune system down. Otherwise, it attack the body.

2 **Macrophages** quickly recognize the viruses as a foreign threat. They begin destroying viruses by engulfing them.

1 The race is on: **Viruses** try to replicate before the immune system can gear up. Two have already taken over cells in the body.

9 As the viruses are being feated, the body creates **mem** T and B cells that circulate per nently in the bloodstream, ensu that next time, that particular will be swiftly conquered.

Fig. 4-1

The immune system is indeed miraculous. Because of its complexity and efficiency, it usually keeps us free from illness. That's why I could work in an elementary school among children with runny noses and sore throats for fourteen years, only taking three sick days. I'm not unusual; most people do the same, because their immune system allows it. When the immune system is suppressed, however, it cannot do its job properly. Then latent cancer cells (which, apparently, we all have from time to time) can freely multiply.

The Meaning of Stress

To say that long-term, unabated stress can inhibit the immune system is meaningless without making clear what is meant by stress. This is a difficult task because we use the same word to describe two very different concepts. The first is an external event, or stressor. Holmes and Rahe (1967) compiled a rating scale of common events such as divorce, illness, or job loss. They put death of a spouse at the top of the scale, giving it a score of 100 (see Figure 4-2). Interestingly, the list includes items that are quite desirable (graduation, marriage, promotion, vacation). They, also, are stressful. So are some everyday items that are not on the list, such as giving a public speech or taking a final exam. People make a distinction between the two types of events, calling the latter "positive stress."

As if that's not confusing enough, we also use the word to refer to our internal reaction to those external events. That's what we mean when we say a person is "stressed out." That's why people write books and teach courses on stress reduction. It is not the event itself, but our reaction to it, that is so significant.

SOCIAL READJUSTMENT RATING SCALE

EVENT	VALUE
Death of a spouse	100
Divorce	73
Marital separation	65
Jail term	63
Death of close family member	63
Personal injury or illness	53
Marriage	50
Fired from work	47
Marital reconciliation	45
Retirement	45
Change in family member's health	44
Pregnancy	40
Sex difficulties	39
Addition to family	39
Business readjustment	39
Change in financial status	38
Death of a close friend	37
Change to different line of work	36
Change in number of marital arguments	35
Mortgage or loan over $10,000	31
Foreclosure of mortgage or loan	30
Change in work responsibilities	29
Son or daughter leaving home	29
Trouble with in-laws	29
Outstanding personal achievement	28
Spouse begins or stops work	26
Starting or finishing school	26
Change in living conditions	25
Revision of personal habits	24
Trouble with boss	23
Change in work hours, conditions	20
Change in residence	20
Change in schools	20
Change in recreational habits	19
Change in church activities	19
Change in social activities	18
Mortgage or loan under $10,000	17
Change in sleeping habits	16
Change in number of family gatherings	15
Change in eating habits	15
Vacation	13
Christmas season	12
Minor violation of the law	11

Figure 4-2: Common Stressors (Holmes and Rahe, 1967)

Take, for example, two different people whose spouse dies. In both cases they had been happily married, so the loss is very great and the suffering is very deep. But in one case the surviving spouse soon begins to count his/her blessings, cultivate old friendships, pursue hobbies, and get involved in community affairs. The other spouse simply despairs, seeing no point in living. The second person's health is at risk, and the future may follow the pattern described poignantly by a friend of mine who said, "My father died fifteen years ago. My mother started dying that same night, but it took seven years."

Thus it is not the external event, but our internal interpretation of it that can lead to suppression of the immune system. Various researchers have shown that anxiety about the future or feeling loss of control causes increased production of adrenaline; prolonged anger stimulates excess excretion of norepinephrine; and feeling overwhelmed or believing that problems are beyond our control increases levels of cortisol (Justice, 1988). As our thoughts and feelings are registered in the brain, signals are sent to secrete the respective stress hormones which, when accumulated in excess, inhibit the immune system and make us vulnerable to illness.

So the ancients were right. There is a relationship between emotions and health. The mind is a powerful force that can help us or hurt us. The fact that we can use this information to our benefit is an incredible source of hope.

PART III

Singing Your Own Song

5

Developing A Positive Outlook

$\mathcal{T}$HE COMMON ELEMENT IN THE CASES described by the early investigators (Galen to Freud) was not a particular event, such as loss of a loved one or undergoing economic hardship, but the feelings that followed: hopelessness and helplessness. Then came the illness. Yet others who experienced the same tragedies did not suffer the same emotional trauma. Why not? Simply because they assessed the situation differently. As was elaborated in Chapter 4, we now know that chronic stress in the form of unresolved negative feelings can stimulate the overproduction of stress hormones and neurotransmitters, which in turn can suppress the immune system, thereby making us vulnerable to illness. The cause, however, is not the external event but the internal interpretation of it. As others have put it, we can't control what happens to us in life, but we can control how we perceive and respond to it. Therein lies the key.

Expectations

We've heard about self-fulfilling prophesies. Children who are frightened at the prospect of playing in a piano recital or adults who are excessively worried about giving a public speech say to themselves, consciously or unconsciously: "I can't do it." "I'll forget." "It won't turn out right." "I'll flub it up." Lo and behold, that's exactly what happens. Those who see the tasks as a challenge they are capable of meeting, prepare themselves as best they can, and believe they will do well, usually are successful.

The same principle can be applied to our health. Remember Ruth, who said she would never get cancer? Of course such a statement didn't determine her destiny, but for sixty years her belief freed her from the anxiety and fear of whether and when she would be diagnosed. In addition, she did everything she could to keep in good health, including drinking raw milk. I am not recommending raw milk to the reader, but I am pointing out that active participation in "wellness" can help make it happen.

Norman Cousins observed the same phenomenon when he was ten years old. As described in *Head First: the Biology of Hope* (1989), Cousins had been living at the time in a tuberculosis sanitorium. He noticed that both children and adults separated themselves into one of two groups: the realists and the optimists. Those in the first group kept to themselves, accepted their "fate," and waited for it to run its course. The others, knowing that it is possible to survive tuberculosis, made friends, laughed, had snowball fights, and read books under the covers by flashlight. In other words, they believed and acted as though they would get well. Many of them did.

A significant study related to this topic was done by Kobasa on "hardiness." After the break up of AT&T, 200 executives at Illinois Bell Telephone were studied. Although they were quite accustomed to dealing with such serious problems as budget, personnel, and public relations, they were in uncharted territory when it came to divestiture. The executives varied greatly in their responses to the break up; so did their subsequent health. Those who felt doomed and without recourse feared the future and acted accordingly. Their bodies got the message, and soon they were sick with various illnesses. Those who saw divestiture as an obstacle that could be overcome went on with normal living and maintained their usual health (Kobasa, 1979).

Visualization

In the treatment of life-threatening illness, beliefs are especially important. There is a significant difference between undergoing treatment with the hope that it will be successful versus truly believing and actively participating to make it so. Although the difference in attitude or approach is psychological, the difference in outcome is physical.

A technique that is especially beneficial is visualization. Athletes use it by picturing their performance in every detail before an event takes place. The value of visualization as a supplement to medical treatment was hinted at in previous chapters, but one of the most impressive examples of its early use and success is found in *Getting Well Again* (Simonton, *et al.*, 1978). The patient was a 63-year-old man with advanced cancer of the throat. His tumor was so large that it affected his ability to swallow, and he had lost significant weight. Radiation was being considered simply to ease the pain of swallowing during his remaining days. Dr. Simonton explained to the patient how the mind can affect the body and the importance of fighting rather than giving up. The man was not only receptive to the idea but eager to try it. Simonton taught him how to use visualization to picture the radiation reducing the size of the tumor. The man did the exercise three times a day for 5 to 15 minutes before and during the radiation treatments. The tumor shrank, the man regained his appetite, he gained weight and lived nine years.

Even after treatment has been completed, visualization can be used to strengthen the immume system. Gruber, *et al.* (1988), worked with metastatic cancer patients for a year, using relaxation and guided imagery. The patients experienced measurable, improved immune functioning, *i.e.*, increased production of antibodies and interleukin-2 cells, enhanced NK-cell activity and improved effectiveness of cytotoxic T cells (Cousins, 1989).

The Will To Live

Using visualization as just described, or even doing something as simple as what I did with my "special sunshine," sets you apart from the passive let-life-happen-to-me point of view, enabling you to try to influence the outcome. Dramatic use of this principle was demonstrated by Norman Cousins and later described in his book *Anatomy of An Illness* (1979). Fifteen years earlier he had been hospitalized with ankylosing spondylitis, a severe degenerative disease of the connective tissue. As he realized that the treatment was ineffective and he was getting progressively worse, he insisted on knowing what the odds were statistically for being cured. He was told 1 in 500. Incredibly, his response was, "What can I do to be that one?" After extensive research on the subject he came up with a program of megadoses of vitamin C, elimination of certain medications, megadoses of laughter (because of its physiological as well as psychological benefits), and determination to live. He did.

A recent report (Goleman, 1985) makes the same point with a more common illness. At King's College Hospital in London, women who had early stage breast cancer treated with a mastectomy were interviewed three months after the surgery. Unbeknownst to them, they were then categorized into four groups, based on their response to the survey questions. The groups were:

1) hopeless, helpless — "I'm as good as dead."
2) stoic acceptance — "Keep a stiff upper lip. Don't complain."
3) denial — "I don't believe I really ever had cancer."
4) fighting spirit — "I'm going to conquer this thing."

Ten years later, statistics were compiled on the 57 women. Survival rates were significantly different among the groups. Only 20% of the hopeless, helpless group and 25% of the stoics were still living. Yet 50% of the deniers were alive, a finding which is interesting to analyze. In psychological circles we say that denial is not helpful or healthful; we're usually talking about denying blame or responsibility for something, however. In the breast cancer study, belief that a specimen was misread in the laboratory and the person never had cancer in the first place is a very beneficial point of view because it totally eliminates any anxiety or fear regarding a reoccurrence, let alone death.

The survival rate in the fighting group was phenomenal: 70%. These statistics show that type and stage of cancer, by themselves, do not determine subsequent progression of the disease. There are other factors involved. Attitude and expectation are among them.

So how can we use this information to help prevent illness or retard its progression? **Believe in ourselves, know that we are worthy and important, and tell ourselves so; realize that our needs are just as important as those of our spouse, our children and our parents; stand up for ourselves as strongly as we do for the underdogs; expect good to come out of adversity; believe that life is worth living, obstacles can be overcome, and there is excitement and meaning to it all.** This philosophy does not guarantee absence of illness, but it contributes significantly to happiness and emotional well being.

Expression of Negative Feelings

The positive outlook just described is an overall philosophy and approach to life in general, as well as to illness in particular. Now that we understand its potential influence on the immunological system, "having a positive attitude" has become the byline of believers of the mind-body philosophy. Well-meaning health professionals tend to emphasize its importance to such an extreme that they risk sending the false message that there is no place for negative thoughts and feelings.

Such a philosophy can be very damaging to our mental and physical health. As chapters 2 and 4 reveal, bottled up negative feelings can prevent the immune system from functioning the way it normally does and make us susceptible to illness. Whether it is grief over the loss of a loved one, anger over being treated unfairly or fear about the future, these feelings need to be recognized and resolved.

A first step is to ventilate your feelings in private. Cry if you need to cry; shout if you need to shout. You'll probably feel better, and that in itself is of value. Next you can tell a sympathetic, supportive relative or friend. Just being heard makes a difference. Many are reluctant to do this, however, for fear of "burdening" someone else with their problems. What a shame that in their greatest hour of need they deny themselves the opportunity to let a friend truly be a friend.

When the issue is anger at someone, the solution is more complex. Ideally one should express that anger directly to the person in a way that can lead to reconciliation, rather than further alienation. Many misunderstandings occur because of misinterpretation of words or behavior. Resolution requires both parties to 1) explain why they did what they did, 2) sincerely apologize for their part, accidental or deliberate, in causing anguish to the other person, and 3) forgive the other person for the anguish he or she caused. Then, and only then, can true reconciliation take place.

The problem is that people are not perfect; everyone does not behave this way. Therefore our anger often continues. We still have other options available, however. One is to write our feelings in a private journal, a process which is known to be therapeutic. Abraham Lincoln is said to have addressed a lot of "people problems" by writing letters which he never mailed. One can also attend a professionally run support group or weekend retreat and ventilate feelings among strangers (which is easier than among friends) or arrange for short-term therapy.

We also have the simple but profound solution of perceiving the situation differently. In other words, what has happened has happened. Nothing can change that. If we are still losing sleep or developing an ulcer because of it, however, then we can choose to assess its meaning or importance differently, in order not to be troubled by it. Thus the positive attitude brings freedom and relief.

There is still a risk of misinterpreting this concept. In Bill Moyer's PBS special "Healing and The Mind," one of the cancer patients in a support group used the phrase, "the prison of positive thinking." She had turned the idea into the simplistic mind-over-matter belief that proper positive thinking could cure illness. If the disease progressed instead, it was because one hadn't exercised adequate mind control (Moyers, 1993).

That concept is a complete misinterpretation of the basic message. **We cannot control our disease any more than we can control any other external event in our life, but we can control the way we interpret and respond to it. Seeing it as a challenge rather than a death sentence, using the warning to make the most of every day, and affirming ourselves as worthy and life as worthwhile can improve the quality of life as long as we live.** That's what it's all about.

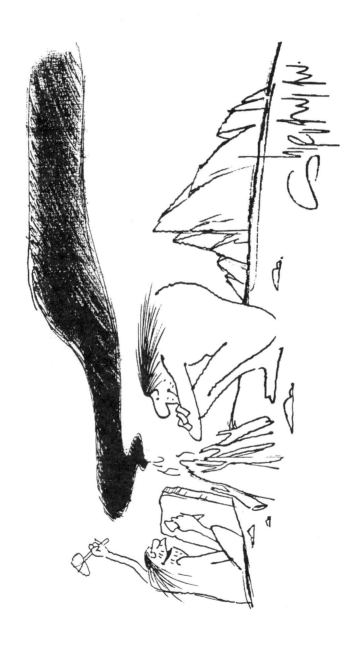

"How do you want to be known in my chronicle, as the discoverer of fire or as the first person to pollute the atmosphere?"

6 ───────────────

Taking Charge

CLOSELY INTERLOCKED WITH ATTITUDE is behavior. Instead of feeling doomed and giving up, we can do the opposite. Replace hopelessness with hope and helplessness with a sense of control. There are several important areas in which to start.

Participation in Decision Making

It is psychologically imperative to actively participate in decision making. In the event of any illness, but especially in a life-threatening one, participation helps negate the feeling of powerlessness and the subsequent negative consequences upon the immune system. Bernie Siegel reminds us that the word patient implies passivity; he prefers to call the person with an illness an "active respant" (Siegel, 1986). At a minimum this means asking questions and getting a second opinion if it may be helpful. Should a physician be irritated or threatened by your approach (like one who said I was trying to "play doctor"), get another doctor.

It is important to feel as comfortable as possible with the doctor, the facility and the treatment. Going a farther distance at a greater expense for treatment is well worth it if you feel more confident about it, but it is not necessary if you feel the same way about your local options. A long-term, positive relationship with your regular doctor may be all you need to feel confident about the recommendations the specialists make. Once you have jointly made the major decisions (regarding such matters as surgery, radiation and chemotherapy), there is still room for your participation in smaller decisions. Years ago a friend of mine did a very daring thing. Prior to her mastectomy she insisted that she be able to listen to classical music on her cassette tape recorder before and during the surgery to keep herself as calm as possible. Wearing ear phones and carrying the machine into the operating room probably broke hospital rules, but her physician acknowledged the far greater importance of her peace of mind and allowed it.

Another example of exerting control comes from a nurse who had had a mastectomy and started chemotherapy. She was hospitalized each time for the treatment. After the first two she decided such caution was unnecessary and the atmosphere was undesirable. She arranged for the rest of the treatments to be given in her doctor's office on an outpatient basis on her way to work. She tolerated the drugs well and experienced minimal hair loss.

What about decision making when you're not sick? It's just as important. Before the women's liberation movement it was typical of many married women to let the man make decisions about such matters as how to spend time, money and vacation. If a woman is truly happy doing that, so be it. If a woman is compromising herself, however, or leaving her needs unmet more of the time than not, it would be better for her mental and physical health to make some changes.

Measurable health benefits of decision making were demonstrated by psychologists Langer and Rodin (1976) in their work with nursing home residents. Starting with the simple task of watering house plants and extending to other responsibilities, they were assigned tasks that had previously been taken care of by staff. Residents who participated in the program showed significant improvement in health within three weeks and had only half the death rate of the controls within eighteen months (Justice, 1988).

Saying No

A few years ago we moved into an old farmhouse that has been in my husband's family since 1882. It was definitely the right move for us, and we have enjoyed slowly renovating, but it is a never-ending job. Before my cancer, if my husband had suggested we start tiling the kitchen some Sunday, I would have agreed without thinking twice about it. Now, because of what I've learned about myself and my needs, I feel free to say no, I'd rather go to church or go for a long walk in the woods or read the *New York Times* from cover to cover.

This is not easy for me to do. The song title "I'm Just A Girl Who Can't Say No" describes my previous pattern of helping people whenever asked. Now I can say no to our daughter about babysitting for a holiday weekend or no to my boss about doing an inservice at a time when I'm already overburdened by other responsibilities. This is of utmost psychological and physiological importance.

The psychiatrist George Soloman raises this difficult question: if we are asked by a friend to do something we really don't want to do, do we say yes or no? If yes, we are compromising ourself and may send a negative signal to our body in the process (Solomon, 1985). Bernie Siegal calls it a "die message," whereas saying no to the friend would be sending a "live message" to our immune system (Siegal, 1986). The point is, if we do too much too often that makes us angry or resentful at ourself or the other person, it can trigger the fight or flight response with the already-described negative effect.

Developing a Support System

Common sense would indicate that social support is important in one's life for a variety of reasons: companionship, an ear to listen to our problems, a sense of feeling wanted and needed, and just having fun. Understandably these benefits build self-esteem and enhance our mental health. But could there possibly be any impact on our physical condition?

Based on his 1959 review of the literature and his own work with cancer patients, psychologist Lawrence LeShan surmised that if loss of a loved one were indeed a significant factor in vulnerability to cancer, then cancer rates should be related to marital status. In other words, widows and widowers should have the highest incidence, then divorcees, and so on down the scale. The validity of his theory was confirmed by statistics from several sources, including those in Figure 6-1, compiled by R. A. Herring from 1929-31 U.S. census data.

single	61.2
married	137.7
divorced	175.8
widowed	527.1

*Figure 6-1: Cancer Mortality Among Women per 100,000 Deaths
(LeShan, 1977)*

Even with a caring spouse in the picture there is value in other kinds of social support, especially when facing a life-threatening illness. National organizations like the American Cancer Society have long sponsored support groups such as Reach for Recovery (for women who have had a mastectomy) and Make Today Count (for cancer patients and their families). Thanks to Harold Benjamin, an accomplished attorney and social psychologist who recognized the need, the Wellness Community was started in Santa Monica, California, in 1982. It provides social, emotional and psychological support for people with cancer, free of charge. The group meets regularly, and participants laugh, cry, get angry, learn about themselves, and inspire each other to take charge. Many of their questions, fears, insights and successes are described in the book *From Victim to Victor*, from which the following is taken:

Stan, a 29-year old accountant who developed brain cancer, is one illustration of how much people can change. When Stan came to The Wellness Community about three years ago, he could hardly walk or talk. Today, because of the fine medical treatment he received, and, he believes, because of his own efforts to recover, only remnants of these infirmities remain. Over several years, Stan spent a great deal of time talking about his personality and the way he reacted to life, and he made some remarkable changes. Before cancer, Stan says he was not proud of himself or happy with life. His immediate reaction to every situation was to think he was not capable of handling it. He was sure he was a failure. But in an appearance on a TV show not long ago, Stan showed a much more positive personality. "I've had three brain operations, chemotherapy, and radiation. I've been through a lot in three years. And all I can say is that because of my experiences with cancer and the fact that my family and friends came through for me, I look at myself completely differently today....I'm actually proud of myself for the first time in many years...and I'm happy with life" (Benjamin, 1987).

Until recently such personal stories were the only evidence we had of the long-term effect of support groups. Understandably, the scientific community wrote them off as anecdotal, but patients and their families believed otherwise. So David Spiegel, a psychiatrist at Stanford University, led a study to investigate. Eighty-six women with metastatic breast cancer were randomly assigned to a support group that met one and a half hours per week or to the control group which did not. All the women received chemotherapy and radiation.

Spiegel was neither hoping nor trying to affect longevity. As he later wrote in Lancet, "We expected to improve the quality of life without affecting its quantity....We intended, in particular, to examine the often overstated claims made by those who teach cancer patients that the right mental attitude will help to conquer the disease" (Spiegel, 1989). He was as surprised as anyone at the results: after being assigned to the support group or the control group, the women who received psychotherapy lived almost twice as long as those who didn't.

Health benefits have also been shown to come from friendship, the most basic kind of social support. Kiecolt-Glaser, et al. (1984) studied thirty elderly people living in retirement homes. When they were visited three times a week for a month, their immune system was enhanced, as measured by improved functioning of antibodies and NK (natural killer) cells (Justice, 1988).

Friendship is also empowering. What is difficult or impossible alone becomes possible and easier with others. Together we can make a difference. As sixteen-year-old Amity Gaige wrote in her national award-winning book:

Individually,
> *we are single drops of rain,*
> *falling silently into the dust,*
> *offering scant promise*
> *of moisture to the thirsty land.*

But, together,
> *we can nourish the Earth*
> *and revive its hopes and dreams.*

Together,
> *we are a thunderstorm.*

(Gaige, 1989)

Setting Goals

A final example of taking charge is to plan for the future. Most would argue that they already do that, buying life and health insurance, managing investments, even doing preventive maintenance on their house or car. What I am advocating, however, is deciding what you want the future to be like and then working toward it. As a school social worker in New Jersey I went into classrooms and ran a program of peer relations. In one session I asked children to write down what they would like to accomplish in the next year. For most, this idea was something they had never thought about, and therefore it was difficult for them to come up with answers. After I gave them examples such as "pass fourth grade" or "make a new friend," they got the idea. I then collected the papers (without names) and compiled their answers into two lists to discuss the following week.

List A was made up of things they had a lot of control over (schoolwork, sports, hobbies and friends); the items on list B were more remote (going to California, getting a horse). We then discussed how to go about trying to accomplish each goal. Even the goals on list B were taken seriously. They led to discussions about earning and saving money, as well as assuming responsibilities in related areas (walking the dog, changing the cat litter) that would make it more likely that their parents might some day consider their wish.

With adults I use a more complex task, modified from a Mid-life Journey weekend conference at Kirkridge, a retreat center in Bangor, Pennsylvania. On a horizontal piece of paper you make four vertical columns, labeling the first column "now" and the fourth column "in five years." You then briefly describe your life at present and what you would like it to be in five years. When I first did the exercise, my first and fourth columns looked like this:

NOW	2	3	IN FIVE YEARS
married			still married
school social worker			have second master's degree & be working in an environmental field
living in New Jersey			find property for building retirement home

Then comes the hard part. Label column 2 as OBSTACLES and column 3 as ENABLING FACTORS. Fill in column 2 with your "excuses" and fears. My anticipated obstacles in going back to school were that I was too old, it would be too difficult and too expensive, there was no one to write a reference twenty years after I'd graduated from college, and I only had a B- average back then anyway.

Surprisingly, however, I came up with the following enabling factors: take one undergraduate science course at a time and get an A, then ask that professor to write a reference for grad school, and use my husband's faculty status to get reduced tuition. I did just that, taking eight courses in three years and getting A's in all but one. Ultimately I chose nutrition rather than environmental science and got the masters at Columbia University. The point is, without having had a goal, I never would have worked toward it.

Given different ages and circumstances, each of us would list different goals. They needn't involve major changes like education or career; they may simply be making more time for friends or starting an exercise program. The important thing, however, is to set goals and work toward them. As Norman Cousins so poignantly put it:

"It is far better to pursue a remote and even unlikely goal than to deprive oneself of the forward motion that goals provide...hope can rekindle one's spirits, create remarkable new energies, and set a stage for genuine growth...regeneration is the greatest force in life...it is not foolish to dream of better things...we discover ourselves as human beings when we move in the direction of our dreams."

(Cousins, 1989)

7

Eating Without Guilt

GOOD NUTRITION BENEFITS us both physically and mentally. A varied, well-balanced diet provides essential ingredients and energy for growth and development. This includes maintenance and repair of cells, tissues and organs as well as biochemical processes such as respiration, circulation and digestion.

Failure of the Four Food Groups

The term *well-balanced* means much more than eating something from each of the basic four food groups. Because of knowledge that has been acquired since that system was devised, what we were taught in elementary school is not adequate. Remember the four groups?

1) milk and dairy products
2) meat, fish, poultry, eggs and nuts
3) fruits and vegetables
4) bread and cereal

We were taught that adults should eat two servings from the milk category, two from meat, four fruits or vegetables, and four servings of bread or cereal per day. The problem is, one can follow those recommendations and still choose nutritionally poor quality foods. The following day's menu makes the point.

Eating a breakfast of apple juice, egg on toast and coffee provides one serving of fruit, one of "meat" and one grain. A lunch of an American cheese sandwich, banana and diet soda provides one dairy serving, two grains and one fruit. Spare ribs, mashed potatoes, green beans, French bread and ice cream for dinner yield one meat, two vegetables, one grain and one dairy. Thus the recommended number of servings has been consumed, but here's what they contain.

	fat (g)	cholesterol (mg)	fiber (g)	calories
breakfast				
apple juice	0	0	1	116
fried egg	7	211	0	91
white toast[1]	1	0	0	55
pat butter	4	11	0	34
lunch				
2 oz. Am. cheese	18	54	0	212
2 pc. white bread[1]	2	0	1	130
banana	1	0	2	105
dinner				
spare ribs	27	107	0	352
mashed potatoes	9	4	3	222
green beans	0	0	2	18
French bread	1	0	1	100
ice cream	14	59	0	269
TOTAL	**84**	**446**	**10**	**1704**

Figure 7-1: Nutritionally Poor Diet from Basic Four Food Groups. (data compiled from food tables in Hamilton, et al., 1991)

[1] A piece of white bread yields about 65 calories, but after being toasted, only 55.

Obviously the day's menu is very high in fat (84 g, which is 44% of total calories[2]), high in cholesterol and low in fiber. It is neither nutritious nor well balanced.

Politics of the Food Pyramid

Realizing the limitations of the Four Food Group system, the USDA did consumer research on this subject and came up with the idea of a food pyramid, which clearly emphasizes the importance of grains, vegetables and fruit and de-emphasizes meat and dairy products. In the spring of 1991 the Eating Right Pyramid was ready for publication but was stopped by opposition from the meat and milk industries (Toufexis, 1991). After another year of research and thousands of taxpayers' dollars, the pyramid was ultimately approved. It is an easily understandable picture of the proper way to eat, not only for general health but also to help reduce the likelihood of heart disease, diabetes, and certain cancers and obesity.

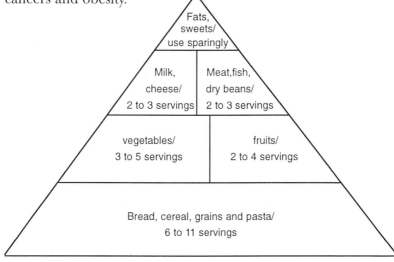

Figure 7-2: Facsimile of Eating Right Pyramid

[2]The term calorie (technically Calorie or kilocalorie) is a measure of heat produced when food is burned in the laboratory. When that same food is digested by the body, the same amount of energy is produced. Some is used to maintain body temperature; some, for processes such as respiration and circulation; some for motion. The rest is saved for future use, stored in the form of fat tissue. Thus we arrive at the layman's understanding of the term: the more calories a food contains, the more "fattening" it is.

It may sound shocking to the reader that 6 to 11 servings of grain are recommended, but a serving is only 1/2 cup or one slice. Thus a cup of cold or hot cereal with toast provides three servings; a muffin or sandwich, two; a cup of potatoes, rice or pasta, two. As much of an improvement as the pyramid is, it has its limitations. We do not need to eat two or three servings from the milk group and two or three from the meat group daily to get the nutrients we need. Furthermore, dried beans and peas (legumes) are listed with meat because they are high in protein, but they are not high in fat, as many meats and meat alternatives are. They are a starchy vegetable and should be listed with the other complex carbohydrates (fruits, vegetables, breads, grains and cereals).

Diet for Good Health

In 1977 the Senate Select Committee on Nutrition determined that our overall daily diet should consist of 12-15% protein, no more than 30% fat, and 55-58% carbohydrates. This principle has been difficult for the non-nutritionist to put into practice. USDA guidelines over the years have helped by talking in terms of minimizing consumption of fat, cholesterol, sugar and salt and increasing consumption of fiber. Now that the pyramid has been published, there is no excuse for claiming ignorance. If we consume the recommended 2-4 servings of fruit, 3-5 servings of vegetables, and 6-11 servings of grain products daily, with occasional servings of lean meat, fish, poultry and dairy products, we will be eating little fat and cholesterol and lots of complex carbohydrates. This is the way of eating that best benefits our health.

The term carbohydrates can be confusing because they include sugar and starch. Sugar, whether it is white, brown, powdered or in the form of honey or corn syrup, is best described nutritionally as "empty calories." In other words, it contains calories (too many of which cause weight gain) without any significant amount of nutrients. A starchy vegetable like lima beans, on the other hand, contains fiber, vitamins and minerals (and far fewer calories than meat or dairy products). Furthermore, complex carbohydrates cause only a slow increase of glucose (or blood sugar) compared to the fast action of sugar.

Many of the fruits and vegetables contain vitamin C, vitamin E, or beta carotene (a substance in plants that our body converts to Vitamin A, as needed). These three vitamins are antioxidants, which are very beneficial to our health. They neutralize free radicals, the unstable, highly reactive molecules that can cause cell damage and contribute to degenerative disease. Many studies have shown that increased consumption of these vitamins is correlated with decreased incidence of cataracts, heart disease and cancer (Godfrey, 1992).

Good food sources of vitamin C include oranges, grapefruit, cantelope, strawberries, broccoli, green peppers and Brussels sprouts. For vitamin E, choose brown rice, whole wheat bread and wheat germ. Beta carotene is found in dark yellow fruits and vegetables such as apricots, cantelope, carrots, sweet potatoes and winter squash. It is also abundant in dark green leafy vegetables, such as spinach and kale. Cruciferous vegetables such as cabbage, cauliflower, broccoli and Brussels sprouts also have antioxidant properties, as does the mineral selenium, which is common in whole wheat, brown rice, dried beans and fish.

Protein is essential for growth and repair of cells, but it can come from plants as well as animals without the usual accompanying fat and cholesterol. In order for the vegetable protein to be complete (*i.e.*, containing all the essential amino acids as meat does), certain combinations must be eaten together or, at least, within the same day. An example is to combine legumes (dried beans or peas) with grains. The Spanish have done this for centuries in their staple of rice and beans; children get the same type of benefit eating a peanut butter sandwich.

To minimize fat consumption one might think that the solution is to become a strict vegetarian, meaning eating no meat, fish, poultry, eggs, milk or milk products like cheese. This is fine if one has strong philosophical or religious beliefs supporting such a regimen and is happy doing so. If not, it can actually have the opposite effect.

When "Good" Can Be Hazardous to Your Health

As a Registered Dietitian and Consulting Nutritionist I am frequently asked for dietary advice. Several years ago a friend called from out of state about her cholesterol level. It was quite high, and she was trying to lower it by diet. She told me about a program run by an M.D. in which participants had actually been able to reduce plaque in their arteries through diet, exercise and stress reduction. The problem was that the diet was so strict (only 10% fat) that it was very hard to figure out what to eat. Shopping and cooking had become a real hassle, and eating was no longer fun. I could tell by her tone of voice and the fact that she was calling for help that she was upset.

"If it's that stressful, stop doing it!" I said emphatically, without knowing anything more about the program than that. Day in, day out frustration and irritation and feeling of failure can trigger the fight or flight response, with all its negative consequences, including raising the cholesterol level which she was trying so hard to lower. I did not end my consultation there. I praised her for her success thus far and wrote a long letter giving her the following suggestions.

Alternatives to Deprivation

High fat foods include many of our favorites: bacon, sausage, croissants, peanut butter, pastrami, pepperoni, spare ribs, cheese, butter, margarine, sour cream and ice cream, to name a few. Reducing fat, however, does not require that we cut out such foods altogether. There are four alternatives:

1) **Eliminate the high fat item(s) in certain dishes.**

   When eating a poached egg on toast, you can do without the butter or margarine without significantly affecting taste. Likewise, pancakes and French toast need only syrup. Plain or mushroom pizza is just as filling and just as much fun to eat as pepperoni, as is meatless lasagne.

2) **Substitute lower fat item(s).**

   Without reducing the quantity of food eaten, one can significantly reduce calories consumed by choosing lower fat items. For example, order tossed salad instead of chef. Snack on popcorn rather than cheese and crackers. Serve frozen yogurt instead of ice cream; drink hot wassail instead of eggnog. For a list of lower fat (and therefore lower calorie) alternatives to some commonly eaten foods, see Figure 7-3.

Instead of:	Choose:	Reducing Intake by:	
		g fat	calories
Danish	English muffin & apple butter	11	47
Scrambled egg with milk, butter	Poached egg	1	16
3 strips of bacon	2 pieces Canadian bacon	5	23
1 cup Cracklin Oat Bran	1 cup Wheaties	8	128
1 cup whole milk	1 cup skim milk	8	64
1 oz. cheddar cheese	1 oz. Mozzarella	4	34
1/2 avocado	1 banana	14	47
1 cup cream chicken soup	1 cup chicken noodle soup	5	40
1 pc. beef bologna	1 pc. ham lunchmeat	4	24
4 choc. chip cookies	5 vanilla wafers	5	87
3 oz. prime rib, lean	3 oz. sirloin steak, lean	10	76
3 oz. broiled salmon	3 oz. poached cod	8	81
chicken drumstick, fried	chicken drumstick, roasted	9	117
2 breaded fish steaks	3 oz. imitation crab	6	68
fried pork chops, lean & fat	broiled pork chops, lean & fat	8	59
1 cake doughnut	40 thin pretzel sticks	9	170
1 piece Boston cream pie	1 piece angel food cake	8	135

Figure 7-3: Comparison of high fat and lower fat foods (data compiled from food tables in Hamilton, et al., 1991).

3) **Eat less of the high fat food.**

A third alternative is simply to cut down on serving size. A grilled cheese sandwich can be made with only one slice of cheese instead of two; likewise a peanut butter sandwich only needs one tablespoon of peanut butter. When tempted by cheese cake in someone's house for dinner, ask for only half a slice.

4) **Eat the high fat food less often.**

In the first weight control class I ever taught, one of my students mentioned that she used two pats of butter on one English muffin. When I suggested that she use half as much butter, she shook her head and said, "I know it won't work. I'll never give up my one pat of butter on each half of my English muffin." Fine. Better to be honest than make false promises. Yet there is still a solution: serve the muffins less often. Instead of eating them five mornings a week, limit them to three.

I would be negligent if I did not say more about the program that my friend found so frustrating. Upon reading the book she had been following (*Dr. Dean Ornish's Program for Reversing Heart Disease*), I found it to be an excellent program of nutrition, exercise and stress reduction. The results speak for themselves: participants showed a measureable decrease in plaque in their arteries (Ornish, 1990).

There is a difference, however, between participating in his study and trying to do the same thing on your own. In the one case, you are part of a group that meets weekly to learn, to try new things, to gripe about what is difficult, and to share what works. There is supervision, social support, inspiration and accountability. It is very different trying to do it alone.

Furthermore, no one knows whether such a restrictive diet (only 10% of calories from fat) is necessary to achieve these results. Considering studies of subcultures within the U.S. in which high fat diets are consumed but incidence of heart disease is low (Hampton, et al., 1964; Stout, et al., 1964; Wolff, 1968), my professional guess is that the exercise and stress reduction components are even more important than the restrictive nutritional one. Chapters 5 and 6 of this book have described some options in these areas; chapters 8, 9 and 10 offer more.

8

Keeping Fit

THERE IS AN OLD CHINESE SAYING that when the student is ready, the teacher will appear. We all know that exercise is good for our health, but most of us need someone or something to jar us into doing it. For some, the diagnosis of a health problem may serve as the impetus; for others, the influence of a friend. For me it was an article in *Social Work* entitled "Running as an Adjunct to Psychotherapy" (Leer, 1980).

Intrigued with the title, I turned to that article in the journal first, wondering how running and psychotherapy could be connected. The author indicated that studies had shown that exercise such as running could trigger the same activity in the brain that would occur as a result of taking antidepressant medication (Greist, *et al.*, 1978). Fascinated with the possibilities for helping others, I turned to the book that people had been raving about for years.

Aerobic Exercise

It was Kenneth Cooper's original book on aerobics (Cooper, 1968) in which he reported his research with more than 5,000 men and women in the U.S. Air Force. To my surprise, in the first few pages I learned that health was more than the absence of illness and that I was not physically fit!

Cooper coined the word aerobics, meaning exercise that causes the body to take in lots of oxygen. Examples are walking, jogging, running, bicycling, swimming and cross country skiing.

Aerobics dance classes and water aerobics were later created by others as alternatives. Achieving the same results depends on intensity of the exercise and frequency of participation.

Cardiovascular Benefits

What Cooper called the "training effect" is the physiological change that takes place in your body after you start doing aerobic exercise on a regular basis. Textbooks now call it cardiovascular conditioning. This includes increased oxygen consumption, increased blood volume, increased strength and stroke volume of the heart, improved circulation, reduced pulse rate, and lowered blood pressure. To achieve these results, one should obtain a doctor's permission to start a gradual exercise program and work up to a minimum of twenty minutes a day, four or five days a week. Cooper and Cooper (1972) and Cooper's later books (1977, 1982) detail specific programs to follow.

Psychological Benefits

The benefits of exercise in terms of cardiovascular conditioning are more widely known than the psychological ones, but it is the latter that can benefit our overall health in terms of the effect of the mind upon the body. When we exercise regularly, we feel happy that we're doing something for ourselves, proud that we're doing something that isn't necessarily fun and takes discipline to do, excited about helping our heart and hopeful about side benefits. So it boosts our self-image and increases our self-confidence. When we do it with another person, we bolster each other's confidence and pride, deepen the friendship, and also have more fun. Cooper summarized the results of his fitness program with the first 5,000 participants as follows:

> In general, most of the diabetics were able to reduce or eliminate medication. The stomach ulcers became less symptomatic. The lung ailments improved. In at least one case, the symptoms of arthritis disappeared, and nearly all of the cardiovascular cases consistently showed improvement.
> The physical rehabilitation, however, was secondary to the personality rehabilitation. This change in their personalities was

manifested by the loss of anxiety and the acquisition of the ability to relax. They had a better self-image and more confidence in themselves. Introverts became extroverts.... The smokers quit or cut down.... The drinkers found that exercise relieved tensions as much as a Manhattan. And, in chorus, they exclaimed they felt better, were more relaxed and were eating less but enjoying it more. The most typical comment was, "I can do more work now with less fatigue, and I sleep like a rock" (Cooper, 1968).

Weight Control

Aerobic exercise is essential for weight control, but twenty minutes at a time is not enough. The reason is that for the first twenty minutes the body burns glycogen. This means the liver converts the stored glycogen back to glucose in order to provide fuel for the extra activity. After about twenty minutes the stored glycogen is used up. Then and only then does the body burn fat. So it is far more effective to exercise for a longer period but fewer times per week. To illustrate this point in classes, I compiled the chart shown in Figure 8-1. There is a significant difference in the benefits of exercising thirty minutes, 5 times a week, versus one hour every other day.

Duration	Frequency	Hrs. exercise, 2 wks.	Hrs. fat burned, 2 wks
30 min	5 days/wk	5 hours	1 hr. 40 min.
1 hour	every other day	7 hours	4 hr. 40 min.

Figure 8-1: Comparison of Amount of Fat Burned in Differing Exercise Schedules

Longevity

In addition to the benefits already described, there is one more reason to start an exercise program: you might live longer. An eight-year study of 13,344 people was done at the Institute for Aerobics Research in Dallas. Participants were initially tested on a treadmill to determine their level of fitness at that time. The end result was that there were two to three times more deaths in the "low fitness" group than in the "moderate fitness" group, irrespective of cause of death (Lemonick, 1989).

When Walking is Not an Option

For most people, walking is the ideal aerobic exercise. It is easy, safe and inexpensive. The only cost is a pair of good walking shoes. So I thought it a good idea to offer a "Wellness Walking" course in my local community to introduce people to exercise, nutrition and stress reduction as a three-fold approach to wellness. Imagine my surprise when three people signed up who had foot or leg problems that prevented them from doing extensive walking. They were willing to pay the full price of the program in order to benefit from only two-thirds of it.

Rather than single out those with physical limitations, I introduced the whole class (and participants in every wellness course I have taught since) to an exercise that can be done sitting down. It is called J'ARM, an activity described in the book by that name (Anderson, 1991). The word was coined from a comment made by a former music conductor who, when asked how he felt when conducting, raved about feeling alive and energetic, "like jogging with the arms." Anderson devised a program of arm exercises by simulating conducting an orchestra, using chopsticks for the baton. Participants can do standard movements or invent their own, as long as they keep moving to the rhythm and have a good time.

The benefits are greater than one would expect. Arm movement increases circulation of blood to the brain because of our physiology. The first branch off the aorta (the artery carrying blood from the heart) subdivides to reach the arm and the head. Thus arm activity brings increased blood supply (with its oxygen and nutrients) to the brain. The stated benefits of J'ARMing are as follows:

- improved heart-lung efficiency
- improved flexibility and balance
- strengthened muscles
- increased level of endorphins[3]
- improved posture
- regulation of weight

(Anderson, 1991)

---

[3] morphine-like substances produced by the body that not only reduce pain but also provide a feeling of well being.

Perseverance

Like a stationary bicycle or a skiing or rowing machine, J'ARMing from a chair has the added benefit of no excuse not to do it. In other words, if it is cold, dark, raining or snowing outside, it doesn't matter. You can still do it. Of course you can also walk, jog or swim on a regular basis if you set your mind to it and plan ahead.

Given our forgetfulness, procrastination, and being "too busy," it helps to be accountable to something or someone. At a minimum, put a card on the refrigerator door to record your efforts. That way a two-day gap will be noticed. Better yet, arrange to do your exercise with someone else. It needn't be the same person every time. You could swim on Tuesday and Thursday with one person, walk on Saturday with another, walk on Sunday with a third. When committed to other people, it is much more likely that you will do it. It is also much more fun.

If you truly care about yourself and your health, you will find a way.

9

Taking Time Out

T HIS CHAPTER could have been titled "Relaxation," but the word means different things to different people. Within the mind-body literature it can refer to specific techniques, such as progressive muscle relaxation, or the end result which they achieve. The latter was named "the relaxation response" by Herbert Benson in his classic book by that title (Benson, 1976). What I mean by "taking time out" is doing anything that diverts one's time and attention away from personal or professional problems and responsibilities.

Progressive Muscle Relaxation

It was the physician Edmund Jacobson who described this technique in his book *Progressive Relaxation*, which was first published in 1929 and reprinted in 1974. The idea came from the realization that emotional stress can produce muscle tension (whether we are aware of it or not) and that physical tension can then contribute to even more emotional anxiety. Thus the practice of deep muscle relaxation benefits us psychologically as well as physically.

Basically the technique consists of getting into a comfortable, relaxed position and focusing on one group of muscles at a time, moving progressively from the feet to the head, or vice versa. You clench or tighten the muscles in that body part for several seconds, consciously feeling the tension involved. Then the muscles are relaxed while you think or whisper that the tension is gone and you feel relaxed. Tape recordings of such thoughts can help. This process should be repeated several times during one sitting and can be done more than once a day. It can be done routinely as a preventive measure or at the time of stress.

Deep Breathing

Another technique is deep breathing. Surprisingly to many, this does not mean loud, fast, inhalation that leads to elevation of the shoulders and expansion of the chest. Proper breathing is done using the diaphragm, the muscle between the ribs and the stomach. The easiest way to practice is to lie down and put your hand on the upper part of your stomach, just below your rib cage. If your stomach rises as you inhale, you are already doing deep breathing. If your chest rises predominantly, however, you are breathing shallowly and not getting all the benefits. Try sniffing to find the location and feel the movement of the diaphragm, then force your stomach up and down as you inhale and exhale. It will take some time and practice to develop the new technique. The value lies in the fact that deep breathing brings more oxygen to the blood and ultimately to body tissues in exchange for the waste product carbon dioxide. Expansion and contraction of the diaphragm enables the lungs to fill and empty more completely. For details on the techniques of muscle relaxation and deep breathing, see Davis, *et al.*, 1988.

Meditation

Having grown up in the Presbyterian Church, I always thought meditation meant reflecting on and praying about a "thought for the day," written by someone else or thought up on my own at a designated time and place for such a purpose. There is value in this, as discussed in the next chapter.

In mind-body circles, however, the word meditation means something very different. It has been practiced by Indian yogis and Zen monks for more than two thousand years and relatively recently has been brought to the West in forms such as Transcendental Meditation. A detailed discussion of the concept comprises one whole chapter of *Mind As Healer, Mind As Slayer* (Pelletier, 1977). For the purpose of introduction, however, it is sufficient to say that this type of meditation does not involve thinking about something but, rather, refraining from thinking about anything else by simply focusing totally on one thing. It can be an object like a flower or the sound of your breathing or a single word or syllable (called a mantra). Examples are the words "peace" or "shalom" or the syllable "om." Complete concentration of attention excludes other thoughts and feelings, including anxious or fretful ones. The end result can be a calming to the point of slowing one's respiration and heart beat, as well as lowering blood pressure.

In the introduction to *Minding the Body, Mending the Mind*, we see how a biologist who previously thought meditation "was for ascetics who lived in caves" turned to it in desperation because of personal and health problems and discovered she could use it to stop oncoming migraine headaches (Borysenko, 1987). Since Benson and Borysenko's founding of the Mind-Body Clinic at the New England Deaconess Hospital (Harvard Medical School), other facilities across the country are now offering courses in meditation to people with chronic pain. For some fifteen years now physicians at the University of Massachusetts Medical Center have referred some of their most difficult cases to Dr. Jon Kabot-Zinn for his eight-week course. What he calls "mindfulness" helps us capture and live in the moment rather than let the "chatter of the mind" run us on "automatic pilot." His philosophy and program are described in his book *Full Catastrophe Living* (1990).

The point for all of us is that by being able to "tune out the world" and achieve a higher level of consciousness or calmness, we can lessen the likelihood of stressors triggering the fight or flight response, with its ensuing negative effect on our health.

Hobbies

There are other ways of taking time out that are important but often overlooked. A hobby, for example, whether it's making something or collecting something, is a diversion from the rest of our life. It's relaxing and fun; it may be educational and may lead to new friends. Focusing on something outside ourselves, especially if it benefits others, can alleviate physical pain, provide more meaning in life, and actually even prolong it. The following stories illustrate these points.

While teaching a week's Elderhostel course on "Emotions and

Health: the Psychology of Well Being," I learned something profound from one of my students. In the morning course on James Joyce, the instructor had asked for volunteers to read parts from one scene in the short story "The Dead." One woman volunteered and did a terrific job. Her tone of voice, her inflections, her feelings were so realistic that all of us got caught up in the drama. She was highly praised by everyone.

After lunch it was time for my class. The woman came early to tell me how the morning's role playing had affected her. For years she had suffered from severe rheumatoid arthritis, and medication did little to relieve the pain. That morning it was so bad that she had considered not coming to class, but she talked herself into it. Then came the opportunity to do what she loves and does so well. She acted with skill, sensitivity and enthusiasm. She threw herself into the part and enjoyed every minute of it. She had every reason to feel satisfied and proud. Now she was coming to tell me that during the reading her pain had gone away and it was only now starting to return. It had been two and one half hours since the "performance."

The other story is about a seventy-one-year-old man who was in the terminal stages of liver cancer. Given his significant deterioration in a short time, his physician estimated that he only had two weeks to live. Lacking family to care for him, he was discharged from the hospital to St. Rose's Home, run by the Hawthorne Dominicans in New York City. He moved in to live his last days in peace and comfort, but the attention and TLC from the staff did wonders. Suddenly life was worth living. There were things he could do and contributions he could make to someone else less fortunate than he. As a former construction worker, he realized he could build dollhouses, even from a wheelchair. He acquired materials and challenged himself to create special effects like moveable windows. When he was featured in *To Live Until We Say Goodbye* (Kubler-Ross and Warshaw, 1978), he had already lived two years.

Pets

Animal lovers know the joy and value of pets. Dogs and cats can be real companions, as well as sources of affection. They can also be lots of fun. Our German shepherd used to play frisbee with us; our cat sends us into gales of laughter when he plays soccer with a marble on our tile floor. For the person living alone, the presence of a pet can be therapeutic. It gives the person something to think about, someone to "do for," and someone to love. Aware of these benefits, some nursing homes have cats in residence, and some hospitals allow pets to be brought in to see a patient. The practice helps in healing.

A friend of ours, two years after his wife died, said emphatically one day, "I'd give anything to have a black lab!" We asked why he didn't get one. He shook his head, saying that he was 73, the dog would probably outlive him, and he wouldn't want to burden his family with finding a home. Knowing he was an active person (still doing downhill skiing), we thought of giving him a dog as a surprise, but we didn't know him that well and were afraid to risk making a mistake.

A year passed, and he brought up the subject again. We knew we had to do something. By calling vets in the area we located a five-month-old female black Labrador retriever. We then called the owner who promptly reduced the price from $200 to $50 when he heard what we wanted to do. With a "go ahead" from our friend's out-of-town son, one Saturday morning we took the dog to Bill.

It was love at first sight. He couldn't stop touching her, and she reciprocated the attention. Overwhelmed, he groped for words, grinning ear to ear while petting her shiny, silky coat. "Oh!...No!...Oh, no...we've got trouble!" he exclaimed, knowing how much he wanted her but fearing it wouldn't work out. After all, his house was thirty feet from the lake on one side and a busy street on the other. Anticipating his concerns, however, we had brought a leash, a twenty-foot lead, and a wire to attach from his house to a tree for the lead to slide on. We said we'd call him in two days and if there were any problem, the owner would take her back.

We had barely gotten home when the phone rang. Bill couldn't wait to tell us that he had gone out and bought "tons of food, two bowls and two books." He was going to take her to the vet on Monday and enroll her in training class in the spring. A few hours later he called back, this time in a very dejected tone of voice. "Susan," he said hesitantly, "I'm sorry to say I've got a real problem." My heart sank. "I've been through every name in the book, and the only fitting one is Susie. Do you mind?"

Within days we heard from other people about the "new Bill." He was out and about, walking and talking, focusing on Susie and forgetting about himself. He called and wrote us periodically about his dear dog and sent us pictures. The story would have happily ended here, but there is another chapter. After seeing that he could form a new relationship, and be happier because of it, six months later Bill got married. Perhaps, just perhaps, Susie helped make that possible.

Music

Whether it's hard rock or heavy metal, country or classic, folk or jazz, music moves us, frees us, and enables us to transcend ourselves. Moving to its rhythm or singing its song are outward expressions of inner reflections of ourselves. The calm, soothing kind can reduce anxiety, and its value is recognized in preparation for surgery. Even without the words being sung, instrumental renditions of "Danny Boy" and "Amazing Grace" elicit or enable tears to flow. Whether it's campers singing "Vive l'amour" or a choir doing the "Hallelujah Chorus" or Bernstein conducting Beethoven's Ninth after the opening of the Berlin Wall, music inspires and uplifts. It also facilitates communication with people who are autistic, mentally retarded or emotionally disturbed. According to Clive Robbins, psychologist and co-director of the Nordoff-Robbins Music Therapy Clinic at New York University, "Music is the one thing that transcends all human emotion" (Barron, 1990).

It can also transcend physical barriers. We had the privilege of seeing Segovia perform at age 90. He was barely able to walk to center stage, even with the assistance of another person. Then he picked up the guitar and was transformed. Nimbly, he strummed and picked as the classical music flowed from his fingers. The audience was spellbound.

Even more amazing is the story Bernie Siegel tells. A man in the terminal stage of cancer revealed that although he had been a successful attorney all his life, he had only gone into the field to please his father. What he had wanted to do was be a musician. So with a life expectancy of less than six months, he quit his practice and took up violin. He loved it. He practiced hard, did well, and three years later was playing in an orchestra.

10

ꟿifting the Spirit

⟲ HEY CAME FROM OREGON, Arizona and Maine. They came with cancer, Parkinson's, MS. Some came to get answers; others, to celebrate life. The one thing they all had in common was hope.

The occasion was a two-day conference on "The Psychology of Illness and the Art of Healing," which I attended in August of 1988. It was led by Bernie Siegel, a New Haven surgeon who works with people with life-threatening illnesses, to help them mobilize their resources for healing. Using the spoken word, art, music, meditation and humor, Siegel integrates body, mind and spirit in his therapeutic approach.

The entire weekend was educational and inspirational, but the highlight for me occurred during the first hour when we participants introduced ourselves. A man named Jerry stood up, somewhat wobbly, and said he had had by-pass surgery six years earlier. While he was in the hospital, he was found to be diabetic. In retrospect, he believed that he had coped well with both conditions. Then a year ago he developed cancer and within ten days was diagnosed with AIDS.

All 150 people listening gasped in unison. He went on to say that by January he was in a wheelchair, waiting to die. "Then somebody gave me Bernie's book," he said confidently, "and I discovered there was something I could do for myself." Within one month he was out of the wheelchair and back to work. Seven months later he was standing there telling us his story.

Even without the opportunity to attend such a conference, we each have several avenues available to lift our spirits.

Laughter

Laughter is one form of having fun, but its value is far greater. As with all "healthy pleasures," the benefits are two-fold: 1) immediate enjoyment and 2) improvement in our health (Ornstein and Sobel, 1989).

It was Norman Cousins who, during his battle with ankylosing spondelitis, discovered that ten minutes of "belly laughter" provided him with two hours of pain-free sleep, without any medication (Cousins, 1978). Miraculous? Not really. We now know that laughter stimulates the release of endorphins, the neurochemicals with properties like morphine. In other words, they provide pain relief and a feeling of euphoria. Because exercise produces similar benefits, Cousins referred to laughter as "internal jogging."

The extent to which Cousins would go to get a good laugh is shown in the famous story that is told about him. In the hospital after a heart attack, Cousins was given a plastic cup for a urine sample. After the nurse left the room, he filled it with apple juice his wife had brought. When the nurse returned to collect the sample, she noticed it was sort of cloudy and commented to that effect. "You're right, it is," he said casually. "Let's run it through again." And he drank it.

Laughter stimulates the thymus gland which manufactures lymphocytes, the white blood cells that help fight off foreign invaders, whether bacteria, viruses or incipient cancers (Justice, 1988). It is in our best interest to do more of it.

We who take life too seriously and are always in a rat race need to take time to look at the funny paper or watch a television comedy or read a humorous book now and then. Figure 10-1 lists some options for reading. Even more important, we should make time to be with friends whom we laugh with and really enjoy. Don't wait for them to call; invite them over. If they live out of state, offer to meet them somewhere for a weekend. Life is too short not to make the most of it.

Books

Title	Author
Without Feathers	Woody Allen
The Rescue of Miss Yaskell & Other Pipe Dreams	Russell Baker
Murphy's Law	Arthur Bloch
Crackers	Roy Blount, Jr.
The Grass Is Always Greener over the Septic Tank	Erma Bombeck
Chocolate: The Consuming Passion	Sandra Boynton
I Never Danced at the White House	Art Buchwald
Dr. Burns' Prescription for Happiness	George Burns
Oh Heavenly Dog!	Joe Camp
Decline & Fall of Practically Everybody	Will Cuppy
The Fourth Garfield Treasury	Jim Davis
The Complete Mother	Phyllis Diller
Dictionary for Yankees	Bill Dwyer
Is It Friday Yet, Luann?	Greg Evans
I Never Met a Kid I Liked	W. C. Fields
Heathcliff Smooth Sailing	George Gately
How to Make Yourself Miserable	Dan Greenburg
Shoot Low, Boys—They're Ridin' Shetland Ponies	Lewis Grizzard
The Blarney Stone American West	John Hewlett
Happy to Be Here	Garrison Keillor
Please Don't Eat the Daisies	Jean Kerr
The Far Side Gallery Two	Gary Larson
The Greatest Shoe on Earth	Jeff MacNelly
The Great Wall Street Joke Book	John Pizzuto
The Reagan Chronicles	Dwane Powell
Rally Round the Flag, Boys!	Max Schulman
Welcome to the Real World	Wes Smith
It's Hard to be Hip Over Thirty and Other Tragedies of Married Life	Judith Viorst
You All Spoken Here	Roy Wilder, Jr.
Mouse Breath Conformity and Other Social Ills	Jonathan Winters

Figure 10-1a: The pick of the belly laughs—books—as selected by the Comprehensive Cancer Center at Duke University

Audiocassettes

Title	Performer
Bloopers	Anonymous
The Ambassador of Goodwill	Jerry Clower
Live in Picayune	Jerry Clower
Top Gum	Jerry Clower
The Best of Bill Cosby	Bill Cosby
Is A Very Funny Fellow, Right!	Bill Cosby
Wonderfulness	Bill Cosby
200 M.P.H.	Bill Cosby
I Don't Get No Respect	Rodney Dangerfield
The Best of W. C. Fields	W. C. Fields
All the President's Wits	Gerald Gardner
The Works	Groucho Marx
News From Lake Wobegon—Winter	Garrison Keillor
Ogden Nash Reads	Ogden Nash
What Becomes a Semi-legend Most?	Joan Rivers
Crackin' Up	Ray Stevens
Surely You Joust	Ray Stevens
He Thinks He's Ray Stevens	Ray Stevens

Videocassettes

Airplane!
All of Me
Back to the Future
Blazing Saddles
Making Mr. Right
Privates on Parade
The Return of the Pink Panther
Silverado
Some Like It Hot
The Making of the Stooges
The Films of Laurel and Hardy
Volunteers

Figure 10-1b: The pick of the belly laughs—audio and video cassettes—as selected by the Comprehensive Cancer Center at Duke University

Love

Love is expressed in many ways: intimacy, passion, caring and companionship. There is also love of self which, if healthy rather than narcissistic, serves to motivate us to do what is good for us, psychologically as well as physically.

One of the best things we can do for ourselves is to help others. While we are listening to, caring about and assisting someone else, we experience the side benefit of feeling wanted and needed. The importance of this is shown in the comments of a friend of mine who has not felt that way since her husband died three years ago.

"I'm still at loose ends," she says. "All my life I took care of my husband, my children, my parents, my grandchildren. Now my husband and parents are gone, and my children and grandchildren don't really need me. I have no one to do for."

No one needs to be in that boat. There are countless people in every community who need our help. Whether it's visiting a shut-in from your church or teaching an illiterate adult to read or planting a garden for a disabled person, the need is there, and organizations are available to connect you.

Hope

We have long understood that hope benefits us psychologically. Being a positive emotion, it makes us feel good, gives us something to look forward to, and replaces negative thoughts and feelings. Now we understand how it helps us physically. Substituting a positive feeling for a negative one enables the immune system to do its job of protecting us rather than be inhibited by overproduction of stress hormones triggered by the fight or flight response. The significance was stressed in Cousins' choice of title for his 1989 book *Headfirst: the Biology of Hope* (emphasis mine).

Faith

Those who believe in a supreme being or higher power find that their faith is a major source of courage and hope. Scripture and prayer can both humble and strengthen; trust can help reduce anxiety and fear. Studies have even shown that people who attend church regularly incur less illness (including depression) than those who go it alone (Comstock and Partridge, 1972; Graham, *et al.*, 1978; Watts, *et al.*, 1985).

Forgiveness

One of the most powerful spiritual concepts in terms of healing is forgiveness. When we have been wronged or treated unfairly and we continue to harbor a grudge, we are the ones who get insomnia and ulcers, not the other person. Forgiving that person frees us to go on living without unnecessary burdens. In like manner, if we have done something we regret (or failed to do something we intended before a loved one died) and we continue to feel guilty, we only hurt ourselves. As Norman Cousins profoundly put it:

I have learned that life is an adventure in forgiveness. Nothing clutters the soul more than remorse, resentment, recrimination. Negative feelings occupy a fearsome amount of space in the mind, blocking our perceptions, our prospects, our pleasures. Forgiveness is a gift we need to give not only to others but to ourselves, freeing us from self-punishment and enabling us to see a wider horizon in life than is possible under circumstances of guilt or grudge.

There are times when we may feel wronged, betrayed, deceived, humiliated. It would be unhealthy not to react against the outrage. But limits need to be set to the emotional punishment such resentments and anger, however justified, can inflict on us...The easiest way to deepen a grievance is to cling to it...Forgetfulness can be an asset in such cases. Forgetfulness is generally regarded as a defect. But forgetfulness allied to forgiveness is a way of erasing the smudges in the mind that come from prolonged brooding over taunts or insults or injustices, real or imagined. Among the prime assets of the human mind is the ability to cut loose from vengeful or burdensome memories (Cousins, 1990).

Wisdom

A friend of mine, Marcia Cowles, wrote a paper in high school on suffering. She noted famous people like Helen Keller and Rembrandt, as well as literary characters such as Telemakhos in *The Odyssey* and David Copperfield in Dickens' novel as having acquired wisdom through suffering. She then described her experience of being in a body cast for two months after hip surgery and the wisdom she acquired from it.

First, I learned the importance of discipline in this world. It took many years of hard work for the doctor to learn just how to cut and mold the hip socket. As a result of his hard work and discipline I will not be crippled later in life. In the moment of need, when the blood clot moved toward my lungs, another doctor knew just what to do. Doctors, nurses, nurse-aides, lab technicians and physical therapists all had to exercise discipline and work hard to learn their skills. Amidst the growing movement of liberation and 'do your own thing,' I learned that there is a place in this world for people of skill and discipline. This, is wisdom.

I also learned that, truly, 'no man is an island.' For three months I was totally dependent, physically and psychologically, on other human beings. Friendly doctors and nurses, friends who came to see me, parents—and one teacher who cared enough to visit me every day, bringing books and good cheer—all meant a great deal to me. I tend to be quite an individualist and a loner. Through this experience I learned that human beings are tied together in a community of mutual needs and support. This, also is wisdom.

Thirdly, I learned compassion. Before the operation I had never been sick and had experienced little physical pain. I thought sick people were weaklings, and I knew nothing of their suffering. Through my experience, a whole new world was opened up to me—a world of pain and illness. I now know the meaning of physical pain and I know what one goes through in a hospital. To be hurt is to begin to know the hurt of others—and this, is wisdom (Cowles, 1970).

Marcia's poignant words are made more so by the fact that she died of bone cancer before age forty. These additional words from her high school paper speak to us as they did to her: "An experience of sorrow, then, can lead to joy. An experience of tragedy can lead to triumph, and an experience of death can lead to renewed life."

It would indeed be wise to occasionally ask ourselves the question that Bernie Siegel asks patients: "If you knew you were going to die tomorrow, what would you do today?" If it would be to answer an unanswered letter or call a friend or resolve a conflict, why not do it now? Another way to phrase it is to say if you knew you only had six months to live, would you keep doing what you're doing, or would you do something else? Without being morbid, adopting a little of this philosophy would result in our prioritizing our values and managing our time so we would do more of what's truly meaningful and brings us joy. This spirit was captured by Nadine Stair, who at age 85 wrote the following:

If I had my life to live over, I'd dare to make more mistakes next time. I'd relax; I'd limber up. I would be sillier than I have been this trip.

I would take fewer things seriously. I would take more chances. I would climb more mountains and swim more rivers. I would perhaps have more actual troubles, but I'd have fewer imaginary ones.

You see, I'm one of those people who lives sensibly and sanely hour after hour, day after day.

Oh, I've had my moments, and if I had it to do over again, I'd have more of them. In fact, I'd try to have nothing else. Just moments, one after another, instead of living so many years ahead of each day.

I've been one of those persons who never goes anywhere without a thermometer, a hot water bottle, a raincoat, and a parachute. If I had to do it again, I would travel lighter than I have.

If I had my life to live over, I would start barefoot earlier in the spring, and stay that way later in the fall. I would go to more dances. I would ride more merry-go-rounds. I would pick more daisies.

(Stair, 1992)

Conclusion

$\mathcal{M}$Y PURPOSE IN WRITING THIS BOOK was threefold: 1) to introduce the idea to some people and clarify it to others that our emotions do affect our health; 2) to provide highlights of the historical evidence and scientific explanation of the mind-body connection; and 3) to offer opportunities for thinking, feeling and behaving in ways that reduce the chance of invoking the fight or flight response, instead boosting the immune system and, thereby, minimizing our susceptibility to illness.

I would do the reader a great disservice, however, to stop without mentioning that some people mistakenly interpret these data to mean that people who get sick are somehow at fault for their illness. Nothing could be further from the truth, and nothing could be more hurtful than to imply that meaning to someone else.

I do not blame myself (or the Board of Education that cut my job by two thirds) for my cancer. I did not do anything that I knew at that time was hazardous to my health. What I have said is that I later learned that bottling up anger, resentment and jealously for years and not standing up for yourself can trigger the fight or flight response, with its subsequent overproduction of stress hormones and neurotransmitters, with the result that the immune system can be suppressed, thereby making a person more susceptible to illness.

This new knowledge or awareness does not bring a burden of guilt; it does just the opposite. It brings 1) an opportunity for developing different coping styles, 2) hope that those styles will be beneficial in terms of improving one's quality of life, and 3) healing, whether physical or emotional or both.

In *Who Gets Sick,* Justice writes: "Recognizing that mind and body are one—with the evidence clearly showing that each constantly affects the other—is not blaming the victim but acknowledging that disease is multidetermined, and the mind cannot be ignored as an influence" (Justice, 1988).

Remember the relief and elation I felt when I stood up for myself three years after I was treated unfairly? I also experienced pride and satisfaction in "playing lawyer" when I made the case for the value of my work, *successfully* persuading the Board to grant me the leave of absence.

Why let our unconscious anxieties, griefs and fears hurt us when we can consciously use our minds to help? **We can help free our immunological systems to do what they are designed to do when we maintain a positive outlook, express negative feelings, recognize and address our own needs as well as those of others, participate in decision making, say "no" some of the time, practice visualization, set goals and work toward them, develop a social support system, deepen our spiritual one, exercise regularly, eat responsibly, and take time out to laugh, love, forgive, relax and have a good time.**

That's truly singing your own song.

References

Ader, R. and N. Cohen. "Behaviorally Conditioned Immuno Suppression," *Psychosomatic Medicine*, 37 (1975), 333-340.

Ader, R., D. Felten and N. Cohen (eds.). Psychoneuroimmunology. San Diego: Academic Press, Inc., 1981.
_____. *Psychoneuroimmunology*. San Diego: Academic Press, Inc., 1991.

Amussat, J.Z. "Quelques Reflexions Sur La Curabilite du Cancer," read at the Academie de Medecine, November 21, 1854.

Anderson, Dale L. *J'ARM For The Health Of It*. Minneapolis: CompCare Publishers, 1991.

Barron, James. "The Songs Of Therapy," *New York Times Good Health Magazine Supplement* (October 7, 1990), 24-58.

Benjamin, Harold H. *From Victim to Victor: For Cancer Patients and Their Families*. New York: Dell Publishing, 1987.

Benson, Herbert. *The Relaxation Response*. New York: Avon Books, 1976.

Borysenko, Joan. *Minding the Body, Mending the Mind*. New York: Bantam Books, 1987.

Cannon, Walter B. *The Wisdom of the Body*. New York: W. W. Norton and Company, 1939.

Comstock, G.W. and K. B. Partridge. "Church Attendance And Health," *Journal of Chronic Diseases*, 25 (1972), 665-672.

Cooper, Kenneth H. *Aerobics.* New York: Bantam Books, Inc., 1968.

_____. *The Aerobics Program For Total Well-being.* New York: Bantam Books, Inc., 1982.

_____. *The Aerobics Way.* New York: Bantam Books, Inc., 1977.

Cooper, M. and K. H. Cooper. *Aerobics for Women.* New York: Bantam Books, Inc., 1972.

Cousins, Norman. *The Anatomy Of An Illness As Perceived By The Patient.* Toronto: Bantam Books, Inc., 1979.

_____. *Head First: The Biology Of Hope.* New York: E.P. Dutton, 1989.

Davis, M., E. R. Eshelman and M. McKay. *The Relaxation And Stress Reduction Workbook.* Oakland: New Harbinger Publishers, Inc., 1988.

Felten, David L. "A Personal Perspective On Psychoneuroimmunology," in Ader, R., *et al.* (eds.), *Psychoneuroimmunology.* San Diego: Academic Press, Inc., 1991, 1117-1120.

_____, S. Y. Felten, S. L. Carlson, J. A. Olschowka and S. Livnat. "Noradrenergic And Peptidergic Innervation Of Lymphoid Tissue," *Journal of Immunology,* 135 (1985), S755-S765.

Gaige, Amity. *We Are A Thunderstorm.* Kansas City: Landmark Editions, Inc., 1989.

Godfrey, Jodi. "Growing Old Healthfully: Are Antioxidants the Answer? " *Enviromental Nutrition,* (January 1992), 1-3.

Goleman, Daniel. "Strong Emotional Response To Disease May Bolster Patient's Immune System," *New York Times* (October 22, 1985), C-1.

_____ and J. Gurin (eds.). *Mind Body Medicine.* Yonkers: Consumer Reports Books, 1993.

Graham, T. W., B. H. Kaplan, J. C. Cornoni-Huntley, S. A. James, C. Becker, C. G. Hames and S. Heyden. "Frequency Of Church Attendance And Blood Pressure Elevation," *Journal of Behavioral Medicine,* 1 (1, 1978), 37-43.

Greer, S., T. Morris and K. W. Pettigale. "Psychological Response To Breast Cancer: Effect On Outcome," *Lancet,* II (1979), 785-87.

Greist, J. H., *et al.* "Antidepressant Running: Running As Treatment For Non-psychotic Depression," *Behavioral Medicine,* 5 (June 1978), 24.

Gruber, B. L., N. R. Hall, S. P. Hersh and P. Dubois. "Immune System And Psychologic Changes In Metastatic Cancer Patients While Using Ritualized Relaxation And Guided Imagery: A Pilot Study," *Scandinavian Journal of Behavior Therapy,* 17 (1988), 25-46.

Guillemin, Roger. "Peptides In The Brain: The New Endocrinology Of The Neuron," *Science,* 202 (4366, 1978), 390-402.

Guy, Richard. *An Essay on Scirrhous Tumours and Cancers.* London: W. Owen, 1759.

Hamilton, E. M. N., E. N. Whitney and F. S. Sizer. *Nutrition Concepts and Controversies.* St. Paul: West Publishing Company, 1991.

Hampton, J., C. Stout, E. Brandt and S. Wolf. "Prevalence Of Myocardial Infarction And Reinfarction And Related Diseases In An Italian American Community," *Journal of Laboratory and Clinical Medicine,* 61 (1964), 866.

Holmes, T. H. and R. H. Rahe. *Schedule of Recent Experience (SRE).* Seattle: Department of Psychiatry, University of Washington School of Medicine, 1967.

Jacobson, Edmond. *Progressive Relaxation.* Chicago: University of Chicago Press, 1974.

Justice, Blair. *Who Gets Sick?* New York: Jeremy P. Tarcher, Inc., 1988.

Kabat-Zinn, Jon. *Full Catastrophe Living: Using the Wisdom of Your Body and Mind to Face Stress, Pain and Illness.* New York: Delta, 1990.

Kiecolt-Glaser, J., R. Glaser, D. Williger, G. Messick, S. Sheppard, D. Ricker and S. C. Romisher. "The Enhancement Of Immune Competence By Relaxation And Social Contact." Paper presented at the annual meeting of the Society of Behavioral Medicine, Philadelphia, May, 1984.

Kobasa, Suzanne C. "Stressful Life Events, Personality And Health: An Inquiry Into Hardiness," *Journal of Personality and Social Psychology,* 37 (1, 1979), 1-11.

Kowal, Samuel J. "Emotions As A Cause Of Cancer," *The Psychoanalytic Review,* 42 (3, 1955), 217-227.

Kubler-Ross, E. and M. Warshaw. *To Live Until You Say Goodbye.* Englewood Cliffs: Prentice Hall, 1978.

Langer, E. J. and J. Rodin. "The Effects Of Choice And Enhanced Personal Responsibility For The Aged: A Field Experiment In An Institutional Setting," *Journal of Personality and Social Psychology,* 34 (1976), 191-198.

Leer, Frederic. "Running As An Adjunct To Psychotherapy," *Social Work,* 25 (1, 1980), 20-25.

Lemonick, Michael D. "Take A Walk-And Live." *Time* (November 13, 1989), 90.

LeShan, Lawrence. "Psychological Studies As Factors In The Development Of Malignant Disease: A Critical Review," *Journal of the National Cancer Institute,* 22 (1, 1959), 1-18.

_____. *You Can Fight for Your Life: Emotional Factors in the Treatment of Cancer.* New York: M. Evans and Co., 1977.

_____. *Cancer As A Turning Point.* New York: Penguin Books, 1989.

Moyers, Bill. *Healing And The Mind.* New York: Doubleday, 1993.

Ornish, Dean. *Dr. Dean Ornish's Program for Reversing Heart Disease.* New York: Random House, 1990.

Ornstein, R. and D. Sobel. *Healthy Pleasures.* Reading, Massachusetts: Addison-Wesley Publishing Company, Inc., 1989.

Paget, J. *Surgical Pathology.* London: Langman's Green, 1870.

Parker, Willard. *Cancer: A Study of Three Hundred Ninety-seven Cases of Cancer of the Female Breast, With Clinical Observations.* New York: Putnam, 1885.

Pelletier, Kenneth. *Mind As Healer, Mind As Slayer.* New York: Dell Books, 1977.

Pert, C. B., G. Pasternak and S. H. Snyder. "Opiate Agonists And Antagonists Discriminated By Receptor Binding In The Brain." *Science,* 182 (4119) (1973), 1359-1361.

Schally, A.V. "Aspects Of Hypothalamic Regulation Of The Pituitary Gland," *Science,* 202 (4363, 1978), 18-28.

Scharrer, E. and B. Scharrer. *Neuroendocrinology.* New York: Columbia University Press, 1963.

Selye, Hans. *The Stress of Life.* New York: McGraw-Hill Book Co., 1956.

Siegel, Bernie. *Love, Medicine and Miracles.* New York: Harper and Row, 1986.

Simonton, O. C., R. Henson, and B. Hampton. *The Healing Journey.* Toronto: Bantam Books, 1992.

Simonton, O. C., S. Matthews-Simonton and J. L. Creighton. *Getting Well Again.* Toronto: Bantam Books, 1978.

Snow, H. *Cancer And The Cancer Process.* London: J and A Churchill, 1893.

_____. *Clinical Notes On Cancer.* London: J and A Churchill, 1883.

_____. *The Reappearance ("Recurrence") Of Cancer After Apparent Extirpation.* London: J and A Churchill, 1870.

Solomon, George. "The Emerging Field Of Psychoneuroimmunology With A Special Note On AIDS," *Advances* 2 (1, 1985), 8.

Solomon, G. F. and R. H. Moos. "Emotions, Immunity And Disease: A Speculative Theoretical Integration," *Archives of General Psychiatry,* 11 (1964), 657-674.

Spiegel, D., J. R. Bloom, H. C. Kraemer and E. Gottheil. "Effect Of Psychosocial Treatment On Survival Of Patients With Metastatic Breast Cancer," *The Lancet,* 2(8668, 1989), 888-91.

Stair, Nadine. "If I Had My Life to Live Over I Would Pick More Daisies," in Sandra Haldeman (ed.), book by same title. Watsonville, California: Papier-Mache Press, 1992.

Stout, C., E. Morrow, E. Brandt and S. Wolf. "Unusual Low Incidence Of Death From Myocardial Infarction: Study Of An Italian American Community in Pennsylvania," *Journal of the American Medical Association,* 188 (1964), 845-49.

Toufexis, Anastasia. "Playing Politics With Our Food," *Time* (July 15, 1991), 57-58.

Wolff, Harold G. *Stress and Disease,* 2nd ed. Revised and edited by Stewart Wolf and Helen Goodell. Springfield, Ill.: Charles C. Thomas, 1968.

Index

A

Ader, R. 21, 22, 75
adrenaline 22, 26
Amussat, J.Z. 14, 75
Anderson, D.L. 56, 57, 75
anger 8, 9, 10, 19, 26,
33, 39, 40, 70, 73
antioxidants 49, 76
anxiety 14, 15, 26, 30,
32, 55, 64, 70
attitude 20, 29, 30, 32,
33, 34, 37, 41, 74

B

Barron, J. 64, 75
Benjamin, H. H. 40, 59, 75
Benson, H. 59, 75
blame 32, 73, 74
Borysenko, J. 61, 75
breast cancer .. 14, 15, 32, 40, 41

C

cancer 4, 5, 6, 7, 10, 13,
14, 15, 16, 19, 20, 22, 23, 24,
30, 31, 32, 34, 38, 39, 40, 47,
49, 62, 64, 65, 66
Cannon, W. B. 17, 18, 19, 75
chemotherapy 16, 38, 40, 41
cholesterol.... 46, 47, 48, 49, 50
Cohen, N. 21, 75
Comstock, G. W. 70, 75
control . 7, 26, 29, 34, 37, 38, 42
Cooper, K. H. 53, 54, 55, 76
Cooper, M. 54, 76
Cousins, N. 30,
31, 44, 66, 69, 70, 76

D

Davis, M. 60, 76

depression 14, 15, 70
diabetes 47, 54

E

emotions. 10, 13, 15, 18, 20, 21
endorphins 56, 66
expectations 20, 21, 29, 32

F

fat 46, 47, 48, 49, 50, 52, 55
fear 6, 18, 30, 32, 33, 40,
.... 70, 44
Felten, D. L. 21, 75, 76
fiber 46, 47, 48
fight or flight 17,
18, 39, 50, 61, 69, 73
forgiveness 33, 70, 74
friendship 26, 41, 44, 54, 66

G

Gaige, A. 41, 76
goals 42, 44
Godfrey, J. 49, 76
Goleman, D. 32, 76
Graham, T. W. 70, 77
Greist, J. H. 53, 77
grief 13, 14, 33
Gruber, B. L. 31, 77
Guillemin, R. 21, 77
Gump, F. E. 4,5
Guy, R. 13, 14, 77

H

Hamilton, E. M. 46, 51, 77
Hampton, J. 52, 77
helplessness 29, 32, 37
heart disease 47, 49, 52, 54
Holmes, T. H. 24, 77
hope 10, 14, 19, 21,
26, 37, 41, 44, 54, 65, 69, 73

hopelessness 29, 32, 37
hormones 22, 26, 29
Q
immune system 21,
22, 23, 24, 26, 29, 31, 33, 37,
39, 41, 69, 73
J
Jacobson, E. 59, 78
Justice, B. 21,
26, 38, 41, 66, 73, 78
K
Kabat-Zinn, J. 61, 78
Kiecolt-Glaser, J. 41, 78
Kobasa, S. C. 30, 78
Kowal, S. J. 13, 15, 78
Kubler-Ross, E. 62, 78
L
laughter 30, 32, 40, 65, 66
Langer, E. J. 38, 78
Lawrence 79
Leer, F. 53, 78
Lemonick, M. D. 56, 78
Le Shan, Lawrence 13, 14,
19, 20, 39, 40, 78, 79
longevity 41, 55
loss 7, 9, 10, 14,
15, 19, 24, 26, 29, 33, 38, 39
love 69, 74
lumpectomy 4, 5
M
mastectomy 3, 4, 5, 32,
38, 40
mind-body connection 7, 9,
10, 13, 14, 15, 16, 19, 33, 59,
60, 73
Moos, R. H. 20, 80
Moyers, B. 13, 21, 34, 79
N
neurotransmitters 22, 29, 73
O
Ornish, D. 52, 79
Ornstein, R. 66, 79
P
Paget, J. 14, 79
Parker, Willard 15, 79

Partridge, K. B. 70, 75
Pelletier, K. 60, 79
Pert, C. B 21, 79
psychoneuroimmunology ....
20, 22
psychotherapy 41, 53
R
radiation 4, 5, 6,
16, 20, 30, 31, 37, 38, 40, 41
Rahe, R. H. 24, 77
relaxation 31, 55, 59, 74
Robbins, C. 64
Rodin, J. 38, 78
S
Schally, A. V. 21, 79
Scharrer, B. 20, 79
Scharrer, E. 20, 79
self image 54, 55
Selye, H. 19, 21, 79
Siegel, B. 37, 38,
39, 64, 65, 72, 79
Simonton, O. C. .. 10, 20, 31, 80
Snow, H. 14, 15, 80
Sobel, D. 66, 79
Solomon, G. 20, 38, 39, 80
Spiegel, D. 41, 80
Stair, N. 72, 80
Steinberg, J. 7, 9, 10
stress 7, 19, 22, 24, 25, 26,
29, 50, 52, 56, 60, 61, 69,73
Stout, C. 52, 80
susceptibility 10, 22, 33, 73
T
Toufexis, A. 47, 80
U
visualization 10, 20, 30, 31
vitamins 32, 48, 49
W
Warshaw, M. 62, 78
wellness.................... 30, 40, 56
will to live 20, 21, 31, 32
Wolff, G. 52, 80

Additional copies of
SINGING YOUR OWN SONG
by Susan Dinklage Multer
may be ordered by sending a check or
money order for $10.95 postpaid for
each copy to:

Distinctive Publishing Corp.
P.O. Box 17868
Plantation, FL 33318-7868
(305) 975-2413

Quantity discounts are also available
from the publisher.